The Vibrant Alkaline Diet Lunch Cookbook

Fast and Cheap Recipes to Enjoy Lunchtime and Boost Your Metabolism

I0145933

Bella Francis

contained within this document, including, but not limited to, — errors, omissions, or inaccuracies.

Table of contents

Healthy Carrot Muffins

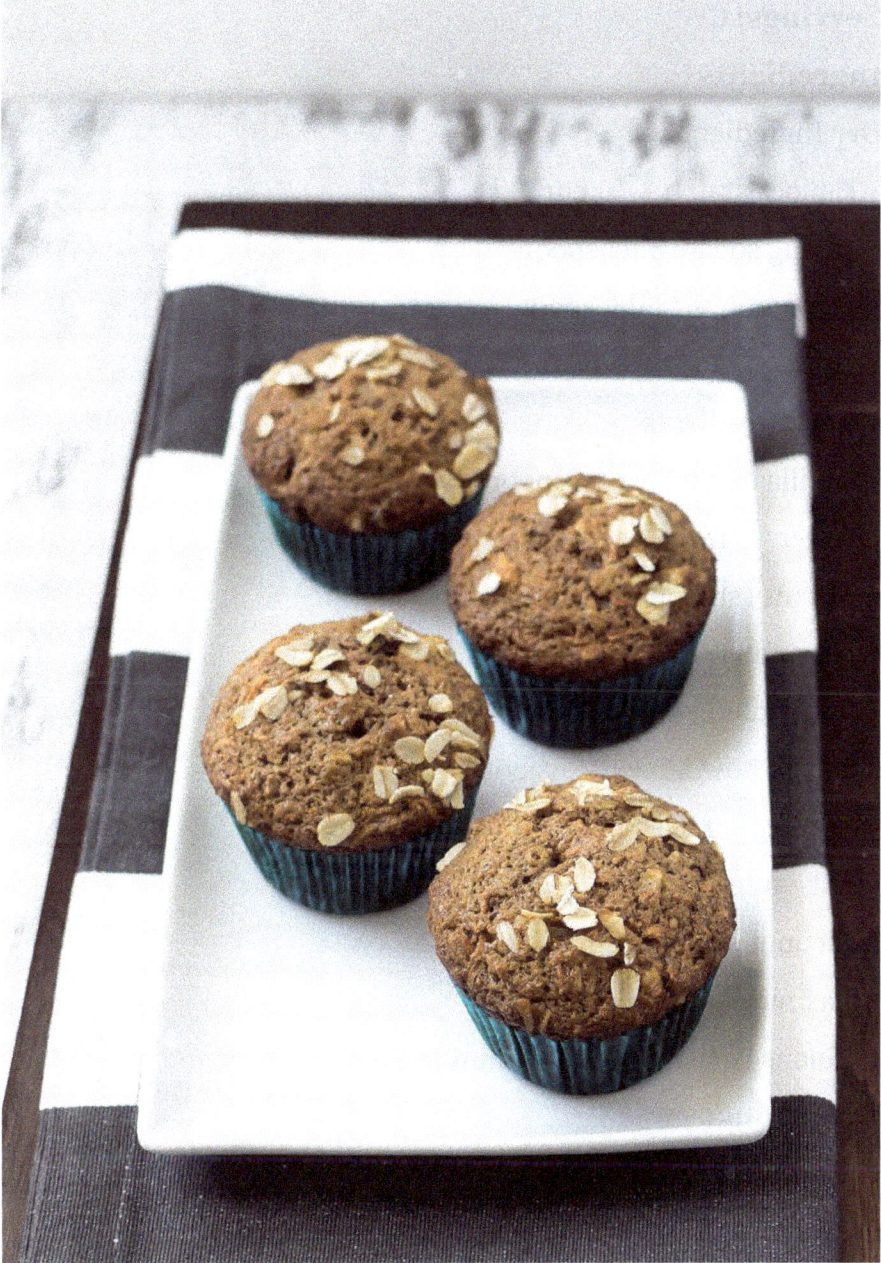

Preparation Time: 10 minutes

Cooking Time: 40 minutes

Servings: 8

Ingredients :

Dry Ingredients

• Tapioca starch – ¼ cup

• Baking soda – 1 teaspoon

• Cinnamon – 1 tablespoon

• Cloves – ¼ teaspoon

• Wet Ingredients

• Vanilla extract – 1 teaspoon

• Water – 11/2 cups

• Carrots (shredded) – 11/2 cups

• Almond flour – 1¾ cups

• Granulated sweetener of choice – 1/2 cup

• Baking powder – 1 teaspoon

• Nutmeg – 1 teaspoon

• Salt – 1 teaspoon

• Coconut oil – 1/3 cup

• Flax meal – 4 tablespoons

• Banana (mashed) – 1 medium

Directions:

1. Begin by heating the oven to 350F.

2. Get a muffin tray and position paper cups in all the moulds. Arrange aside.

3. Get a small glass bowl and put half a cup of water and flax meal. Allow this rest for about 5 minutes. Your flax egg is prepared.

4. Get a large mixing bowl and put in the almond flour, tapioca starch, granulated sugar, baking soda, baking powder, cinnamon, nutmeg, cloves, and salt. Mix well to combine.

5. Conform a well in the middle of the flour mixture and stream in the coconut oil, vanilla extract, and flax egg. Mix well to conform a mushy dough.

Then put in the chopped carrots and mashed banana. Mix until well-combined.

6. Make use of a spoon to scoop out an equal amount of mixture into 8 muffin cups.

7. Position the muffin tray in the oven and allow it to bake for about 40 minutes.

8. Extract the tray from the microwave and allow the muffins to stand for about 10 minutes.

9. Extract the muffin cups from the tray and allow them to chill until they reach room degree of hotness and coldness.

10. Serve and enjoy!

Nutrition:

Calories: 189 calories per serving

Fat – 13. 9 g

Protein – 3. 8 g

Carbohydrates – 17. 3 g

Vegetable Noodles Stir-Fry

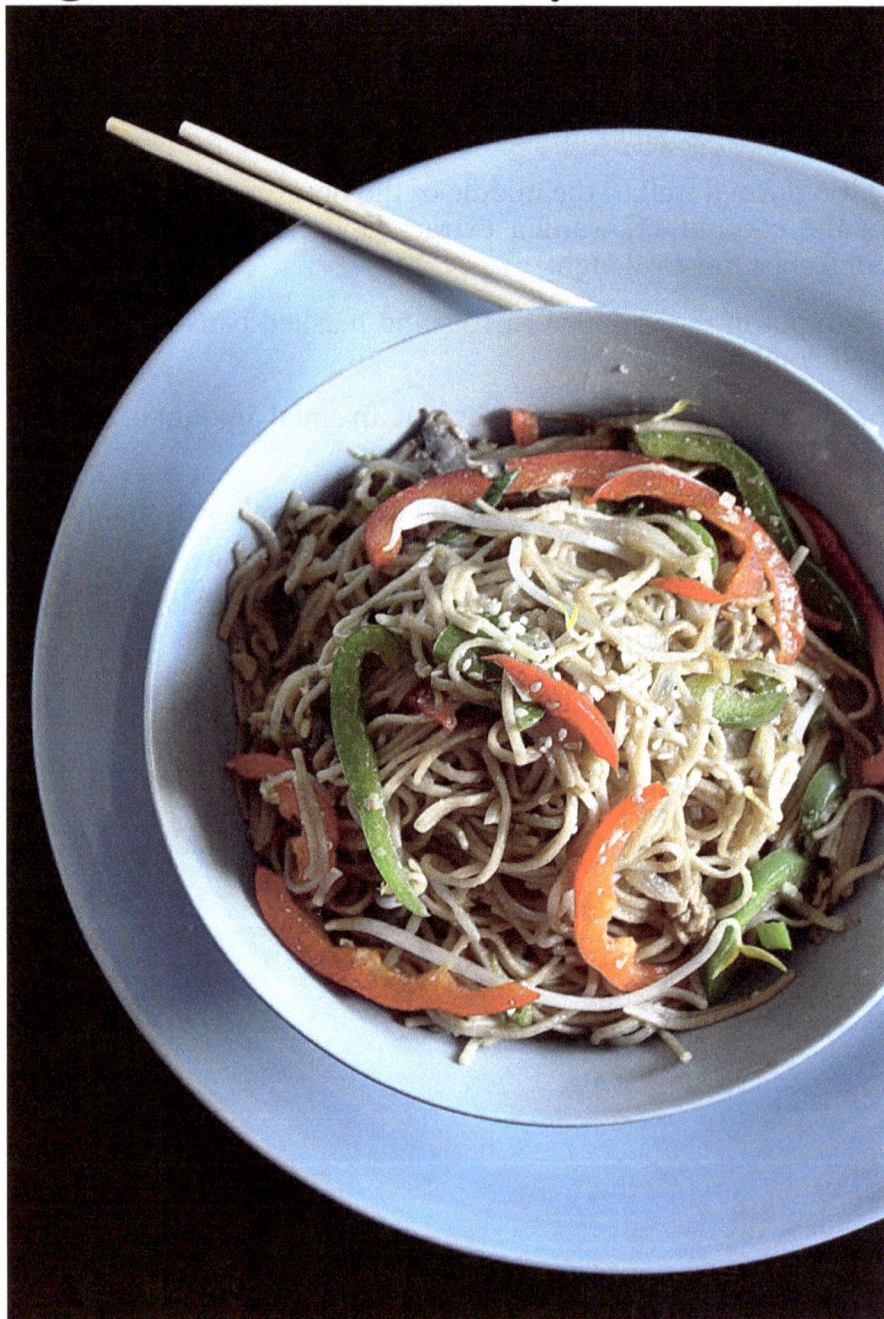

Preparation Time: 10 minutes

Cooking Time: 40 minutes

Servings: 4

Ingredients :

• White sweet potato – 1 pound

• Zucchini – 8 ounces

• Garlic cloves (finely chopped) – 2 large

• Vegetable broth – 2 tablespoons

• Salt – as per taste

• Carrots – 8 ounces

• Shallot (finely chopped) – 1

• Red chili (finely chopped) – 1

• Olive oil – 1 tablespoon

• Pepper – as per taste

Directions:

1. Begin by scrapping the carrots and sweet potato. Make Use a spiralizer to make noodles out of the sweet potato and carrots.

2. Rinse the zucchini thoroughly and spiralize it as well.

3. Get a large skillet and position it on a high flame. Stream in the vegetable broth and allow it to come to a boil.

4. Toss in the spiralized sweet potato and carrots. Then put in the chili, garlic, and shallots. Stir everything using tongs and cook for some minutes.

5. Transfer the vegetable noodles into a serving platter and generously spice with pepper and salt.

6. Finalize by sprinkling olive oil over the noodles. Serve while hot!

Nutrition:

Calories: 169 calories per serving

Fat – 3. 7 g

Protein – 3. 6 g

Carbohydrates – 31. 2 g

Berry-Oat Breakfast Bars

Preparation Time: 10 minutes

Cooking Time: 25 minutes

Servings: 12

Ingredients :

• 2 cups fresh raspberries or blueberries

• 2 tablespoons sugar

• 2 tablespoons freshly squeezed lemon juice

• 1 tablespoon cornstarch

• 11/2 cups rolled oats

• 1/2 cup whole-wheat flour

• 1/2 cup walnuts

• ¼ cup chia seeds

• ¼ cup extra-virgin olive oil

• ¼ cup honey

• 1 large egg

Directions:

1. Preheat the oven to 350f.

2. In a small saucepan over medium heat, stir together the berries, sugar, lemon juice, and cornstarch. Bring to a simmer. Reduce the heat and simmer for 2 to 3 minutes, until the mixture thickens.

3. In a food processor or high-speed blender, combine the oats, flour, walnuts, and chia seeds. Process until powdered. Add the olive oil, honey, and egg. Pulse a few more times, until well combined. Press half of the mixture into a 9-inch square baking dish.

4. Spread the berry filling over the oat mixture. Add the remaining oat mixture on top of the berries. Bake for 25 minutes, until browned.

5. Let cool completely, cut into 12 pieces, and serve. Store in a covered container for up to 5 days.

Nutrition:
calories: 201;
total fat: 10g;
saturated fat: 1g;
protein: 5g;
carbs: 26g;
sugar: 9g;
fiber: 5g;
cholesterol: 16mg;
sodium: 8mg

Sweet and Sour Onions

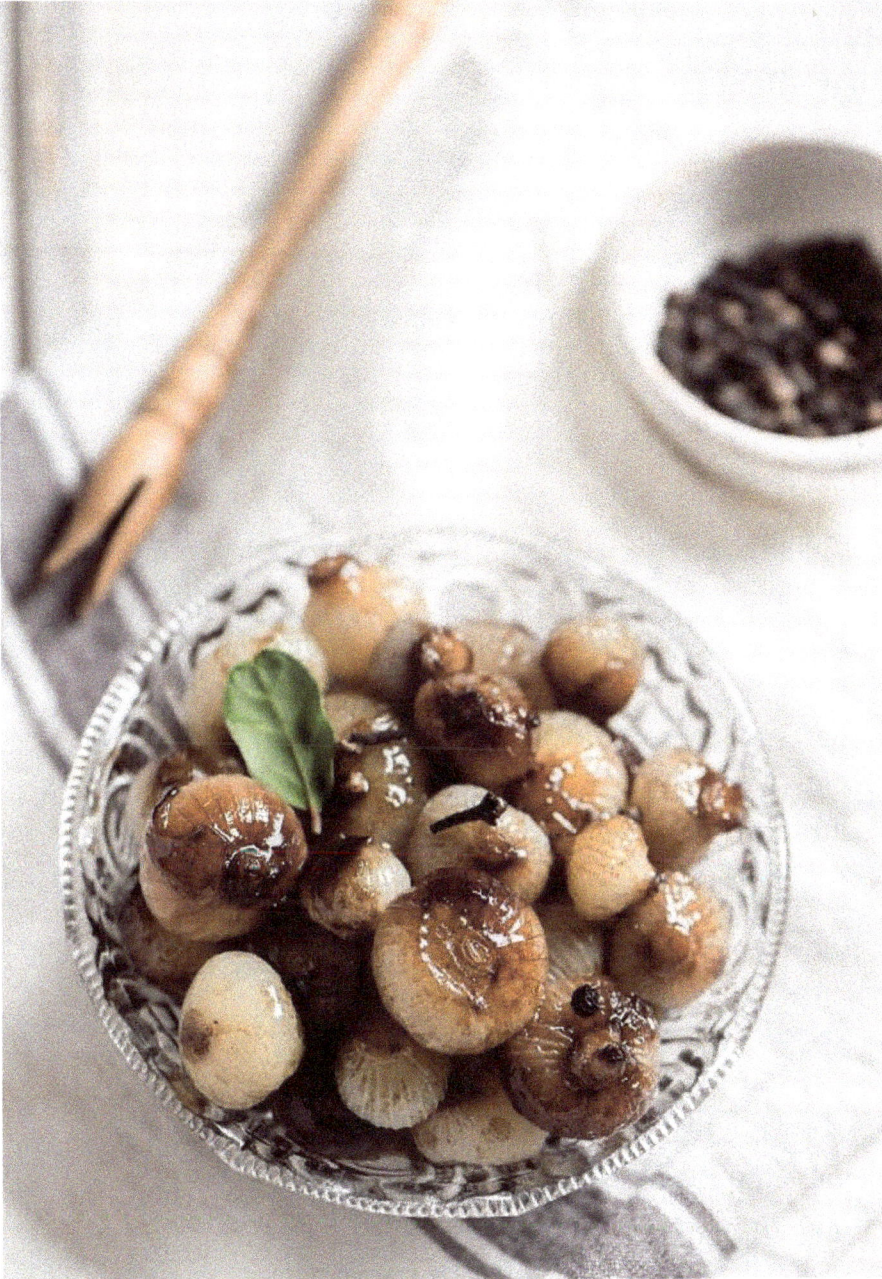

Preparation Time: 10 minutes

Cooking Time: 11 minutes

Servings: 4

Ingredients :

• 4 large onions, halved

• 2 garlic cloves, crushed

• 3 cups vegetable stock

• 1 ½ tablespoon balsamic vinegar

• ½ teaspoon Dijon mustard

• 1 tablespoon sugar

Directions:

1. Combine onions and garlic in a pan. Fry for 3 minutes, or till softened.

2. Pour stock, vinegar, Dijon mustard, and sugar. Bring to a boil.

3. Reduce heat. Cover and let the combination simmer for 10 minutes.

4. Get rid of from heat. Continue stirring until the liquid is reduced and the onions are brown. Serve.

Nutrition:

Calories 203

Total Fat 41. 2 g

Saturated Fat 0.8 g

Cholesterol 0 mg

Sodium 861 mg

Total Carbs 29. 5 g

Fiber 16. 3 g

Sugar 29. 3 g

Protein 19. 2 g

Sautéed Apples and Onions

Preparation Time: 14 minutes

Cooking Time: 16 minutes

Servings: 3

Ingredients :

- 2 cups dry cider

- 1 large onion, halved

- 2 cups vegetable stock

- 4 apples, sliced into wedges

- Pinch of salt

- Pinch of pepper

Directions:

1. Combine cider and onion in a saucepan. Bring to a boil until the onions are cooked and liquid almost gone.

2. Pour the stock and the apples. Season with salt and pepper. Stir occasionally. Cook for about 10 minutes or until the apples are tender but not mushy. Serve.

Nutrition:

Calories 343

Total Fat 51. 2 g

Saturated Fat 0.8 g

Cholesterol 0 mg

Sodium 861 mg

Total Carbs 22. 5 g

Fiber 6. 3 g

Sugar 2. 3 g

Protein 9. 2 g

Zucchini Noodles with Portabella Mushrooms

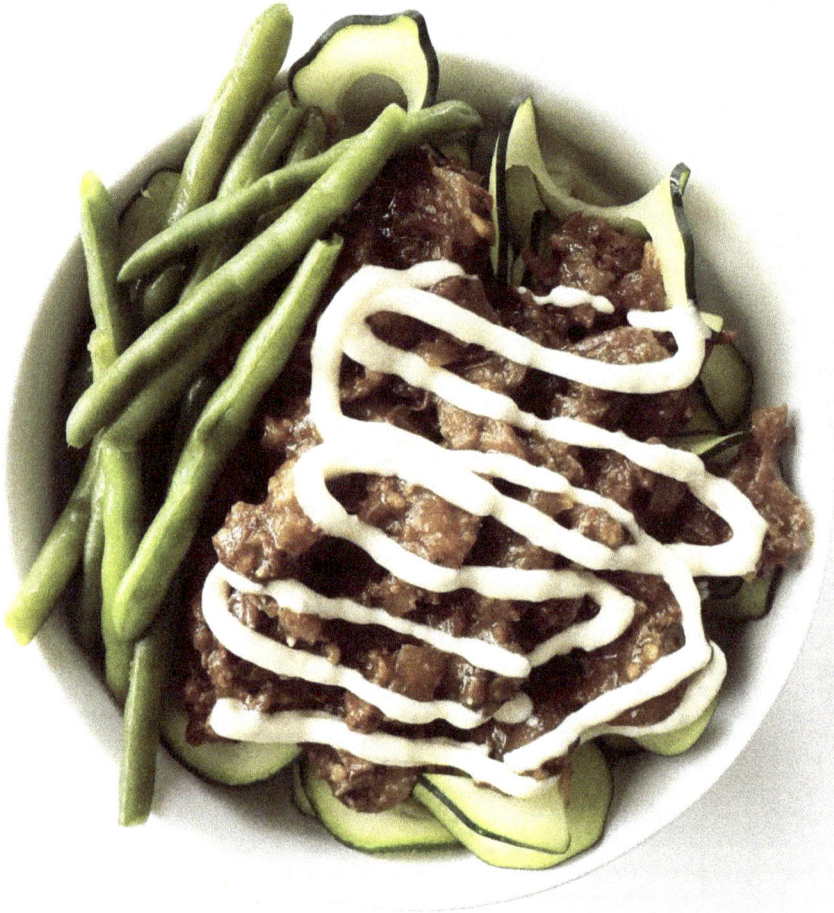

Preparation Time: 14 minutes

Cooking Time: 16 minutes

Servings: 3

Ingredients :

- 1 zucchini, processed into spaghetti-like noodles

- 3 garlic cloves, minced

- 2 white onions, thinly sliced

- 1 thumb-sized ginger, julienned

- 1 lb. chicken thighs

- 1 lb. portabella mushrooms, sliced into thick slivers

- 2 cups chicken stock

- 3 cups water

- Pinch of sea salt, add more if needed

- Pinch of black pepper, add more if needed

- 2 tsp. sesame oil

- 4 Tbsp. coconut oil, divided

- ¼ cup fresh chives, minced, for garnish

Directions:

1. Pour 2 tablespoons of coconut oil into a large saucepan. Fry mushroom slivers in batches for 5 minutes or until seared brown. Set aside. Transfer these to a plate.

2. Sauté the onion, garlic, and ginger for 3 minutes or until tender. Add in chicken thighs, cooked mushrooms, chicken stock, water, salt, and pepper stir mixture well. Bring to a boil.

3. Decrease gradually the heat and allow simmering for 20 minutes or until the chicken is forking tender. Tip in sesame oil.

4. Serve by placing an equal amount of zucchini noodles into bowls. Ladle soup and garnish with chives.

Nutrition:

Calories 163

Total Fat 4. 2 g

Saturated Fat 0.8 g

Cholesterol 0 mg

Sodium 861 mg

Total Carbs 22. 5 g

Fiber 6. 3 g

Sugar 2. 3 g

Protein 9. 2 g

Grilled Tempeh with Pineapple

Preparation Time: 12 minutes

Cooking Time: 16 minutes

Servings: 3

Ingredients :

- 10 oz. tempeh, sliced

- 1 red bell pepper, quartered

- 1/4 pineapple, sliced into rings

- 6 oz. green beans

- 1 tbsp. coconut aminos

- 2 1/2 tbsp. orange juice, freshly squeeze

- 1 1/2 tbsp. lemon juice, freshly squeezed

- 1 tbsp. extra virgin olive oil

- 1/4 cup hoisin sauce

Directions:

1. Blend together the olive oil, orange and lemon juices, coconut aminos or soy sauce, and hoisin sauce in a bowl. Add the diced tempeh and set aside.

2. Heat up the grill or place a grill pan over medium high flame. Once hot, lift the marinated tempeh from the bowl with a pair of tongs and transfer them to the grill or pan.

3. Grille for 2 to 3 minutes, or until browned all over.

4. Grill the sliced pineapples alongside the tempeh, then transfer them directly onto the serving platter.

5. Place the grilled tempeh beside the grilled pineapple and cover with aluminium foil to keep warm.

6. Meanwhile, place the green beans and bell peppers in a bowl and add just enough of the marinade to coat.

7. Prepare the grill pan and add the vegetables. Grill until fork tender and slightly charred.

8. Transfer the grilled vegetables to the serving platter and arrange artfully with the tempeh and pineapple. Serve at once.

Nutrition:

Calories 163

Total Fat 4. 2 g

Saturated Fat 0.8 g

Cholesterol 0 mg

Sodium 861 mg

Total Carbs 22. 5 g

Fiber 6. 3 g

Sugar 2. 3 g

Protein 9. 2 g

Lentil-Stuffed Potato Cakes

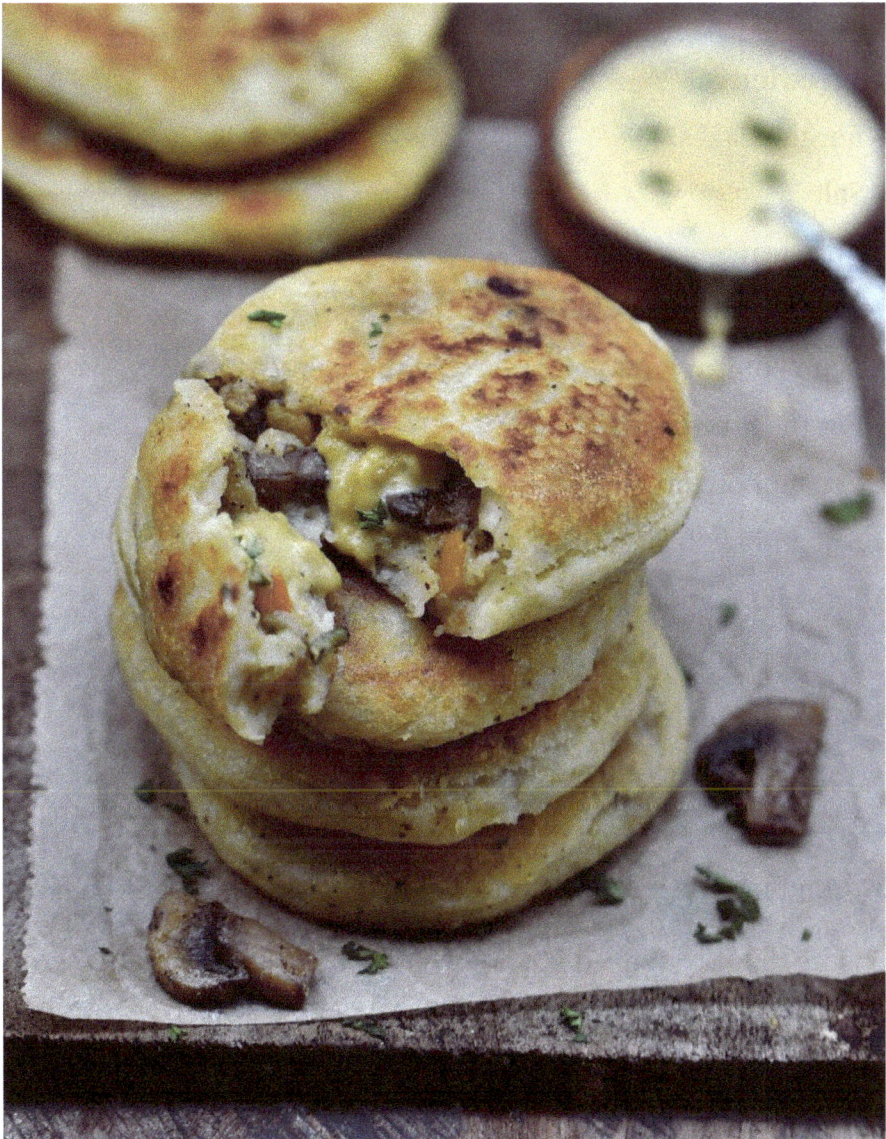

Preparation Time: 15 Minutes

Cooking Time: 30 minutes

Servings: 4

Ingredients

- For the Cakes:
- Salt
- 1 bay leaf
- 10 medium gold potatoes
- 1 cup potato starch- add more for dusting
- For the Stuffing:
- Coconut oil for panfrying
- Salt and freshly ground black pepper
- 1 medium onion, chopped
- 4-ounces mushrooms
- 2 tablespoons olive oil
- ¾ cup dried green lentils (preferably French lentils)- cooked

Directions:

1. Combine the 7 cups of water, potatoes and bay leaf in a large pot and boil until the potatoes are tender. Poke with a fork to ensure they are cooked.

2. Rinse the potatoes under cold water when done; the skins will peel off easily. Now mash the potatoes until smooth and add the potato starch, stir to make dough. Add more potato starch if the dough feels too sticky.

3. For the stuffing, add olive oil to a sauté pan and place over medium high heat. Add in onions and cook as you stir for 5 minutes. Add in the lentils together with pepper and salt (to taste) and cook for 2 minutes. Set aside.

4. To make the cakes, scoop about 3 tablespoons of the dough on your hand and press it into your palm. Add a spoonful of stuffing on top of the dough and fold it over to close it. Shape it into a round disk.

5. Now add coconut oil to a skillet and heat over medium heat. Cook the potato cakes on both sides until golden, roughly 4 minutes per side.

Nutrition:

Calories: 197

Sesame Ginger Cauliflower Rice

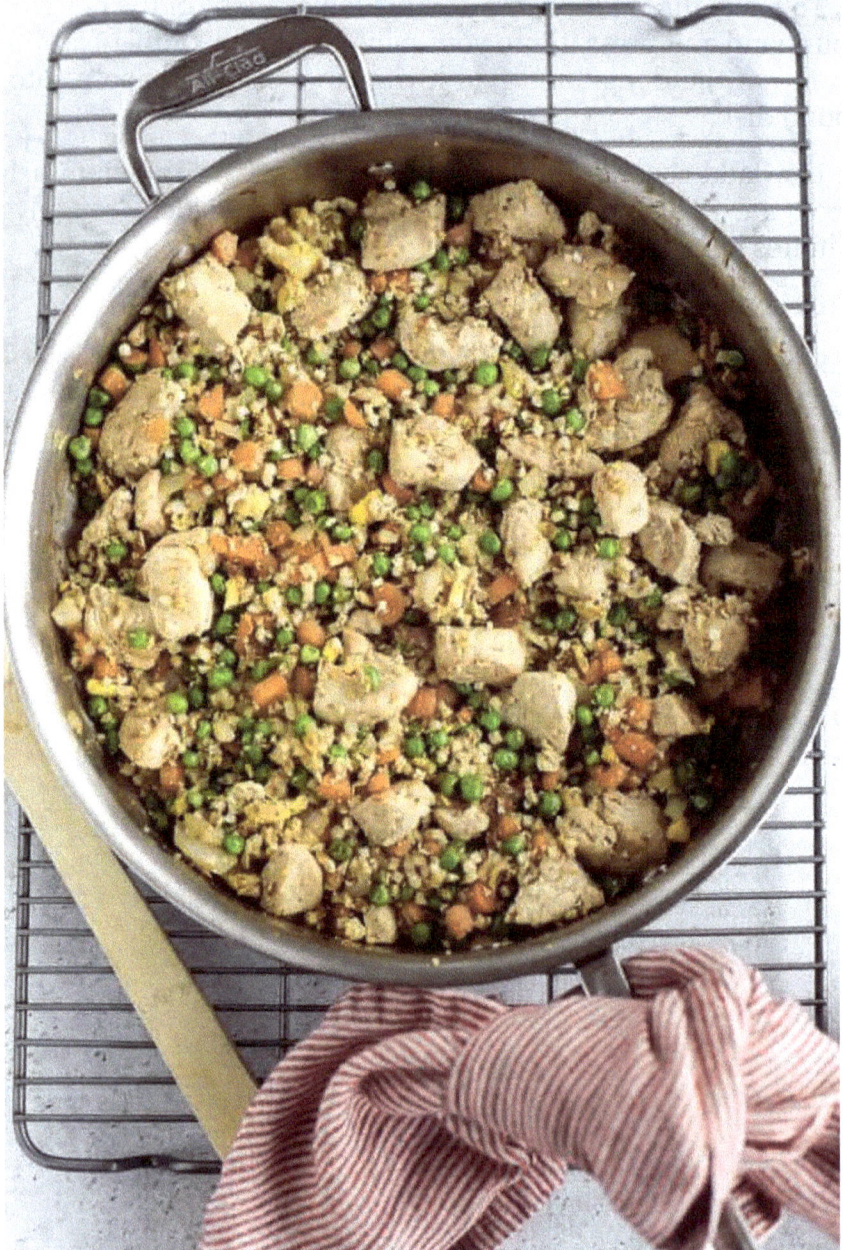

Preparation Time: 10 Minutes

Cooking Time: 15 minutes

Servings: 4

Ingredients

• 2 tablespoons wheat-free tamari plus more to taste

• 4 cups finely chopped mushrooms

• 1 large head cauliflower

• 2 tablespoons toasted sesame oil

• 2 tablespoons grapeseed oil

• 1/2 teaspoon Celtic sea salt- plus more to taste

• 6 green onions- finely chopped (white and green parts)

• 1 bunch cilantro- finely chopped (1/2 cup)

• 2 tablespoons minced fresh ginger

• 2 teaspoons fresh lime juice- plus more to taste

• 1 small green chile- ribbed, seeded, and minced

• 4 teaspoons minced garlic (4 cloves)

Directions:

1. For the cauliflower rice, roughly cut the cauliflower into florets and get rid of the tough middle core.

2. Fit a food processor with an S blade and add the florets to pulse. Pulse for a few seconds until the florets achieve a rice like consistency. You should have 5 to 6 cups of rice in the end.

3. Heat oil in a deep skillet or wok over medium high heat and fry the ginger, green onions, chili, garlic and mushroom seasoned with ¼ teaspoon of salt for 5 minutes. Once combined well and soft, add in the tamari and cauliflower rice and cook for 5 more minutes until soft.

4. Add in remaining salt, cilantro, and lime juice and adjust the flavors as desired.

5. Serve and enjoy!

Nutrition:

Calories: 83

Nori Wraps with Fresh Vegetables and Quinoa

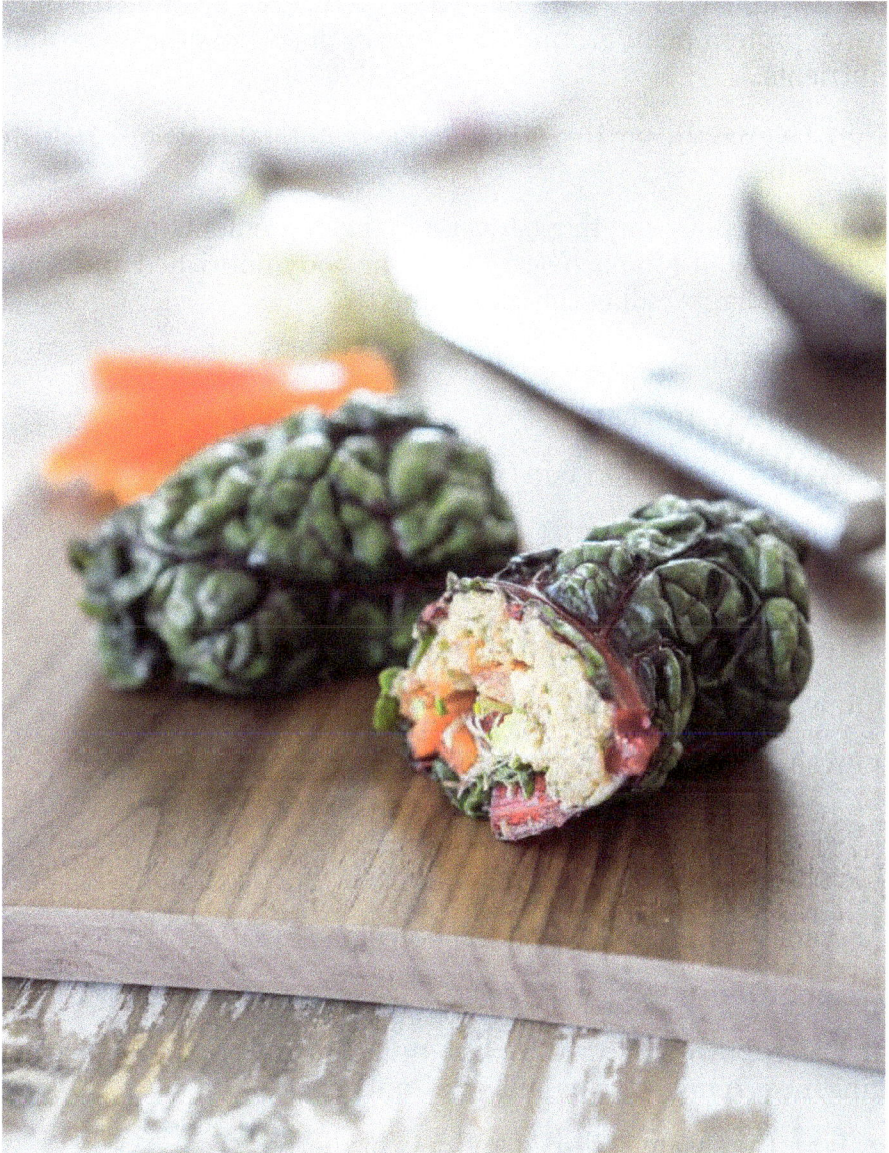

Preparation Time: 15 Minutes

Cooking Time: 20 minutes

Servings: 1

This is an extremely high nutrient alkaline diet for everyone out there. Quinoa, which is a source of protein, is considered the only 100% protein plant around. It is rich in fiber and other essential nutrients.

Nori (seaweed), on the other hand, is antioxidant and rich in nutrients.

When you put everything together, the Ingredients in this diet will leave your stomach satisfied, your body nourished and your taste bud happy, all at the same time.

Ingredients :

• Nori sheets, two (2)

• Raw carrot sticks, ¼ cup (60ml)

• Cooked quinoa, ½ cup (125 ml)

• Raw carrot sticks, ¼ cup (60ml)

• Fresh garlic, finely chopped, one (1) teaspoon (5ml)

• Raw seed mix, one (1) tablespoon (15ml)

• Fresh ginger root, finely grated, one (1) teaspoon (5ml)

• Raw cucumber sticks, ¼ cup (60ml)

• Fresh coriander leaves, finely chopped, ¼ cup (60ml)

• Sesame oilseed, one (1) tablespoon (15ml)

Directions:

1. Get a bowl and mix cooked quinoa with coriander leaves, ginger, seed mix, coriander leaves, and garlic.

2. Pour the sesame oil seed and mix properly.

3. Spread out both nori sheets on two surfaces.

4. Spread the quinoa mix one each nori sheets.

5. Add carrot sticks and cucumber on top of the quinoa.

6. Fold up the nori sheets with the quinoa Ingredients inside.

7. Depending on how you like it, serve with pickled ginger or soy sauce.

Nutrition:

Calories: 160

Kale Wraps with Chili, Garlic, Cucumber, Coriander, and Green Beans

Preparation Time: 30 Minutes

Cooking Time: 0 minutes

Servings: 2

The **Ingredients** that make up this diet are incredibly nutritious to the body. Let's start with Green beans – they are rich in fiber and also serve as a cleansing agent to the colon.

Kale is extremely useful when it comes to detoxifying the body because it helps in cleansing the kidney.

The Avocado and raw seed mix are replete with cholesterol-lowering fat, which is essential in keeping the body healthy.

And Coriander, on the other hand, remains a real source for essential nutrients and fiber.

Now, when you consider everything put together, this meal is highly nutritious, healthy and delicious. The best part is, it's alkaline.

Ingredients :

1. Fresh lime juice (30ml), one (1) tablespoon

2. Raw seed mix (15ml), one (1) tablespoon

3. Kale leaves (large), two (2)

4. Fresh garlic (finely chopped, 10ml), two (2) teaspoons

5. Ripe avocado (pitted and sliced), half (½)

6. Fresh red chili (seeded & finely chopped), one (1) teaspoon (5ml)

7. Fresh cucumber sticks (250ml), one (10) cup

8. Fresh coriander leaves (finely chopped), (125ml), ½ cup

9. Green beans (250ml), one (1) cup

Directions:

1. Spread kale leaves on a clean kitchen work surface.

2. Spread each chopped coriander leaves on each leaf, position them around the end of the leaf, perpendicular to the edge.

3. Spread green beans equally on each leaf, at the edge of each leaf, same as the coriander leaves.

4. Do the same thing with the cucumber sticks.

5. Cut the divide chopped garlic across each leaf, sprinkling it all over the green beans.

6. Cut and share the chopped chili across each leaf and sprinkle it over the garlic.

7. Now, divide the avocado across each leaf, and spread it over chili, garlic, coriander and green beans.

8. Share the raw seed mix among each leaf, and sprinkle them over other Ingredients.

9. Divide the lime juice on across each leaf and drizzle it over all other Ingredients.

10. Now fold or roll up the kale leaves and wrap up all the Ingredients within it.

11. You can serve with soy sauce!

Nutrition:

Calories: 298

Cabbage Wraps with Avocado, Asparagus, Pecan Nuts and Strawberries

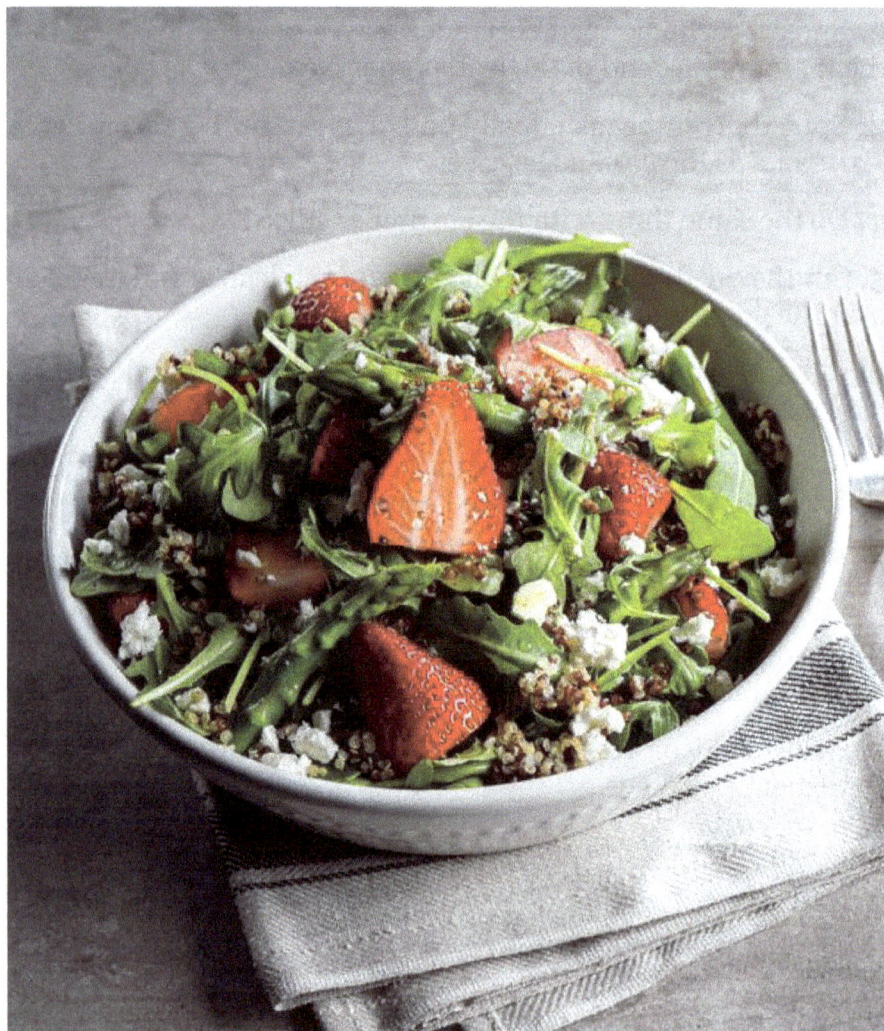

Preparation Time: 30 Minutes

Cooking Time: 0 minutes

Servings: 1

The Cabbage wraps with avocado, asparagus, pecan nuts, and strawberries is another delicious and powerful alkaline diet at your service.

If you are conscious of your health, there is every possibility that you must have heard about the alkaline diet and how it helps stabilize the human body pH. The Ingredients in this meal are super rich in nutrients, e.g., in as much as strawberries are natural sweeteners, they are also anti-oxidants. Asparagus, on the other hand, possess an inherent property that helps mitigate aging. Its ability to help drain the liver is also an impressive feature in the process of detoxification.

It is exceptionally delicious and healthy.

Ingredients :

• Raw pecan nuts (roughly chopped), 125 ml, ½ cup

• Fresh sliced strawberries, 124 ml, ½ cup

• Cabbage leaves, two (2) large

• Ripe avocado (pitted & sliced), ½

• Green asparagus spears (250 ml), one (1) cup

Directions:

1. Spread out the cabbage sheets on a clean kitchen work surface.

2. Share the asparagus shear among each cabbage leaf and place them on the edge of the leaf.

3. Share the avocado slices on each leaf and put them on top of the asparagus spears.

4. Share the strawberries over each leaf and spread on top of the avocado slices.

5. Share the pecan nuts between each leaf and spread it on the strawberries.

6. Wrap the leaves with all Ingredients inside them.

7. Serve with soy sauce (optional).

8. Enjoy.

Nutrition:

Calories: 146

Millet Tabbouleh, Lime and Cilantro

Preparation Time: 15 Minutes

Cooking Time: 20 minutes

Servings: 6

This super alkaline delicacy is tasty, nutritious, and filling. The Ingredients that make up this meal are millet, tomatoes, lime juice, hot sauce, olive oil, green onions, cucumber, and cilantro.

The Millet Tabbouleh, Lime, and Cilantro recipe is guaranteed to keep your blood pH alkaline, which in turn translates to healthy living, productiveness, and happiness.

Enjoy this recipe.

Ingredients :

• Lime juice, ½ cup

• Cilantro (chopped), ½ cup

• Hot sauce, 5-6 drops (Tabasco)

• Olive oil, ¼ cup and two (2) teaspoons (divided)

• Tomatoes (diced), two (2) large

• Green onions, two (2) bunches

• Cucumber (peeled, seeded and juiced), two (2)

• Millet (rinsed and drained), one (1) cup

Directions:

1. Heat olive oil in a saucepan over medium heat.

2. Add the millet and fry until it begins to smell fragrant (this takes between three (3) to four (4) minutes).

3. Add about six (6) cups of water and bring to boil.

4. Wait for about fifteen (15) minutes.

5. Turn off the heat, wash and rinse under cold water.

6. Drain the millet and transfer to a large bowl.

7. Add cucumbers, tomatoes, lime juice, cilantro, green onions, the ¼ cup oil, and hot sauce.

8. Season with pepper and salt to taste.

Nutrition:

Calories: 240

Lemony Salmon Burgers

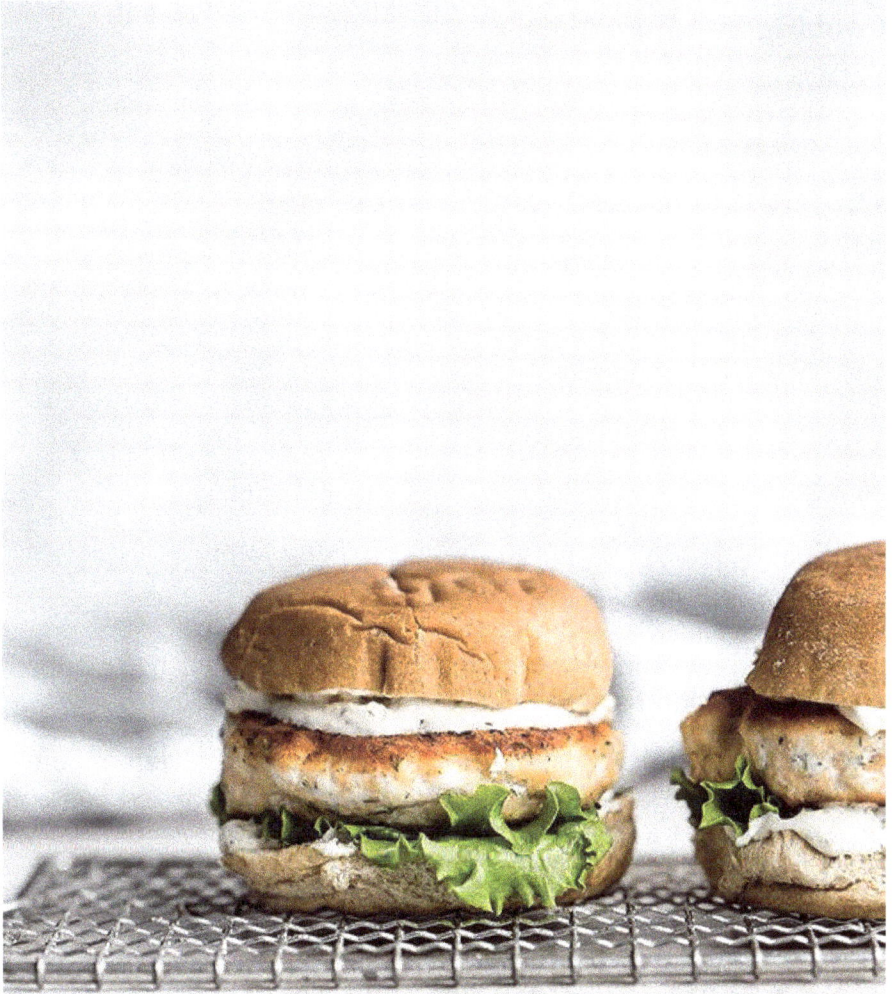

Preparation Time: 10 Minutes

Cooking Time: 10 Minutes

Servings: 4

Ingredients

• 2 (3-oz) cans boneless, skinless pink salmon

• 1/4 cup panko breadcrumbs

• 4 tsp. lemon juice

• 1/4 cup red bell pepper

• 1/4 cup sugar-free yogurt

• 1 egg

• 2 (**1.** 5-oz) whole wheat hamburger toasted buns

Directions:

1. Mix drained and flaked salmon, finely-chopped bell pepper, panko breadcrumbs.

2. Combine 2 tbsp. cup sugar-free yogurt, 3 tsp. fresh lemon juice, and egg in a bowl. Shape mixture into 2 (3-inch) patties, bake on the skillet over medium heat 4 to 5 Minutes per side.

3. Stir together 2 tbsp. sugar-free yogurt and 1 tsp. lemon juice; spread over bottom halves of buns.

4. Top each with 1 patty, and cover with bun tops.

This dish is very mouth-watering!

Nutrition:

Calories 131

Protein 12

Fat 1 g

Carbs 19 g

Caprese Turkey Burgers

Preparation Time: 10 Minutes

Cooking Time: 10 Minutes

Servings: 4

Ingredients

- 1/2 lb. 93% lean ground turkey

- 2 (1,5-oz) whole wheat hamburger buns (toasted)

- 1/4 cup shredded mozzarella cheese (part-skim)

- 1 egg

- 1 big tomato

- 1 small clove garlic

- 4 large basil leaves

- 1/8 tsp. salt

- 1/8 tsp. pepper

Directions:

1. Combine turkey, white egg, Minced garlic, salt, and pepper (mix until combined);

2. Shape into 2 cutlets. Put cutlets into a skillet; cook 5 to 7 Minutes per side.

3. Top cutlets properly with cheese and sliced tomato at the end of cooking.

4. Put 1 cutlet on the bottom of each bun.

5. Top each patty with 2 basil leaves. Cover with bun tops.

My guests enjoy this dish every time they visit my home.

Nutrition:

Calories 180

Protein 7 g

Fat 4 g

Carbs 20 g

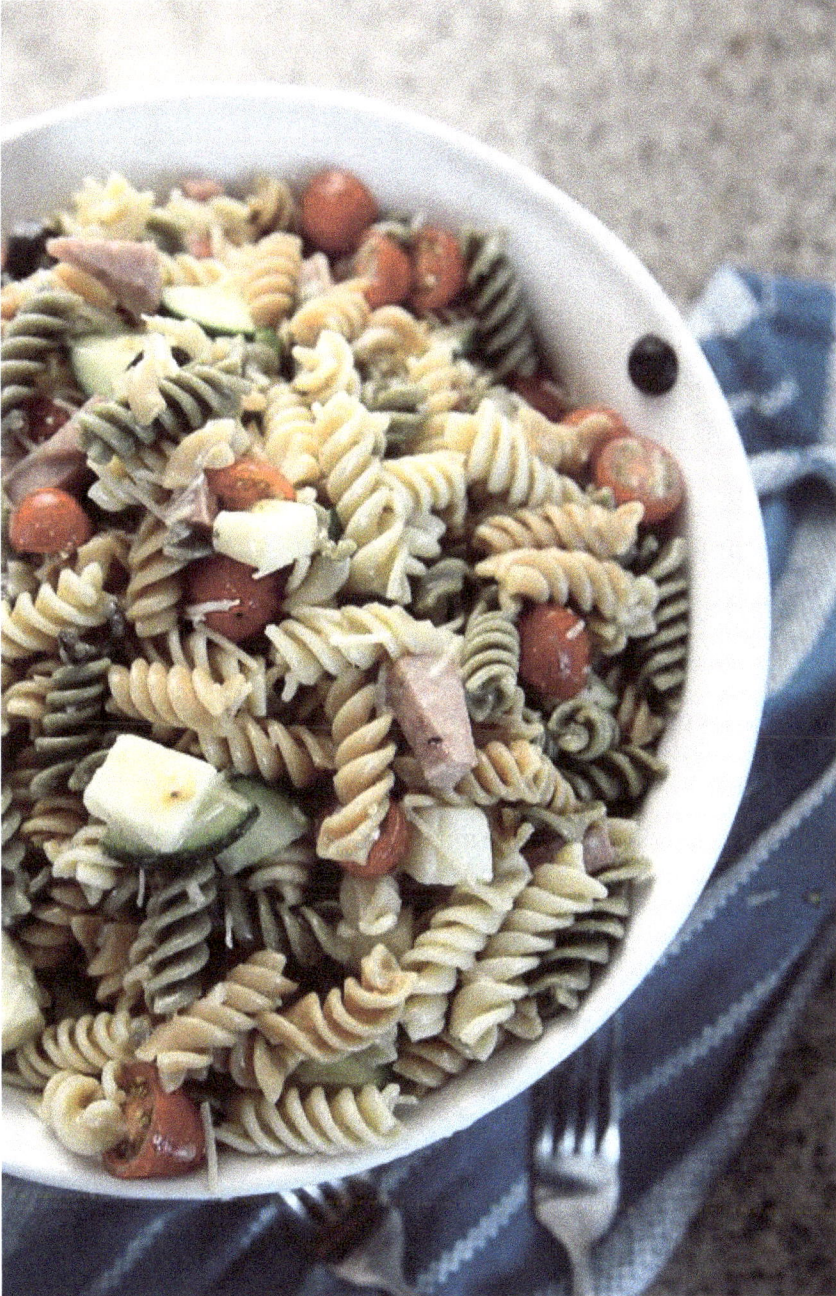

Pasta Salad

Preparation Time: 15 Minutes

Cooking Time: 15 Minutes

Servings: 4

Ingredients

• 8 oz. whole-wheat pasta

• 2 tomatoes

• 1 (5-oz) pkg spring mix

• 9 slices bacon

• 1/3 cup mayonnaise (reduced-fat)

• 1 tbsp. Dijon mustard

• 3 tbsp. apple cider vinegar

• 1/4 tsp. salt

• 1/2 tsp. pepper

Directions:

1. Cook pasta.

2. Chilled pasta, chopped tomatoes and spring mix in a bowl.

3. Crumble cooked bacon over pasta.

4. Combine mayonnaise, mustard, vinegar, salt and pepper in a small bowl.

5. Pour dressing over pasta, stirring to coat.

Understanding diabetes is the first step in curing.

Nutrition:

Calories 200

Protein 15 g

Fat 3 g

Carbs 6 g

Lemon-Thyme Eggs

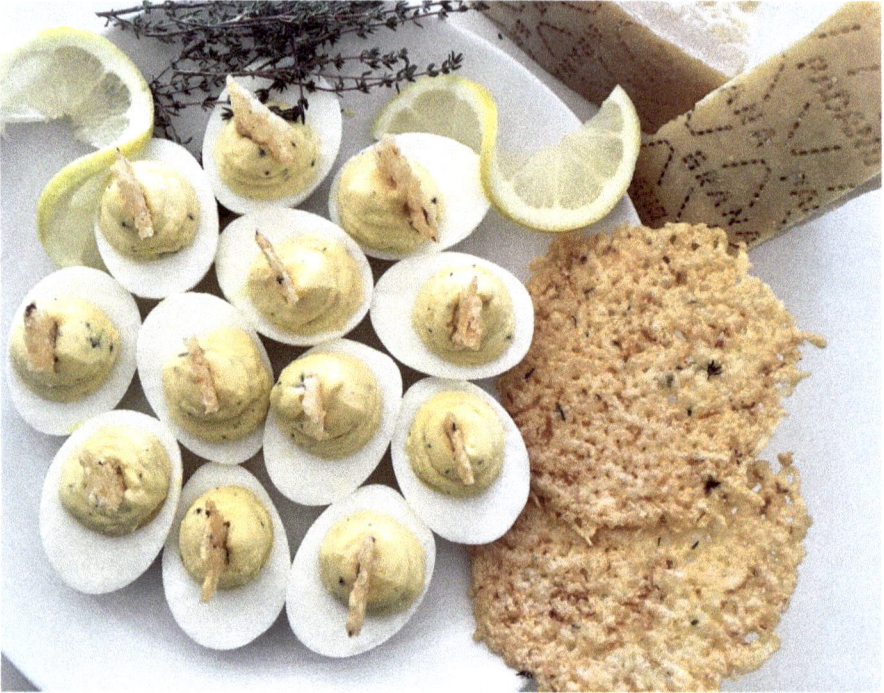

Preparation Time: 10 Minutes

Cooking Time: 5 Minutes

Servings: 4

Ingredients

- 7 large eggs
- 1/4 cup mayonnaise (reduced-fat)
- 2 tsp. lemon juice
- 1 tsp. Dijon mustard
- 1 tsp. chopped fresh thyme
- 1/8 tsp. cayenne pepper

Directions:

1. Bring eggs to a boil.

2. Peel and cut each egg in half lengthwise.

3. Remove yolks to a bowl. Add mayonnaise, lemon juice, mustard, thyme, and cayenne to egg yolks; mash to blend. Fill egg white halves with yolk mixture.

4. Chill until ready to serve.

Please your family with a delicious meal.

Nutrition:

Calories 40

Protein 10 g

Fat 6 g

Carbs 2 g

Spinach Salad with Bacon

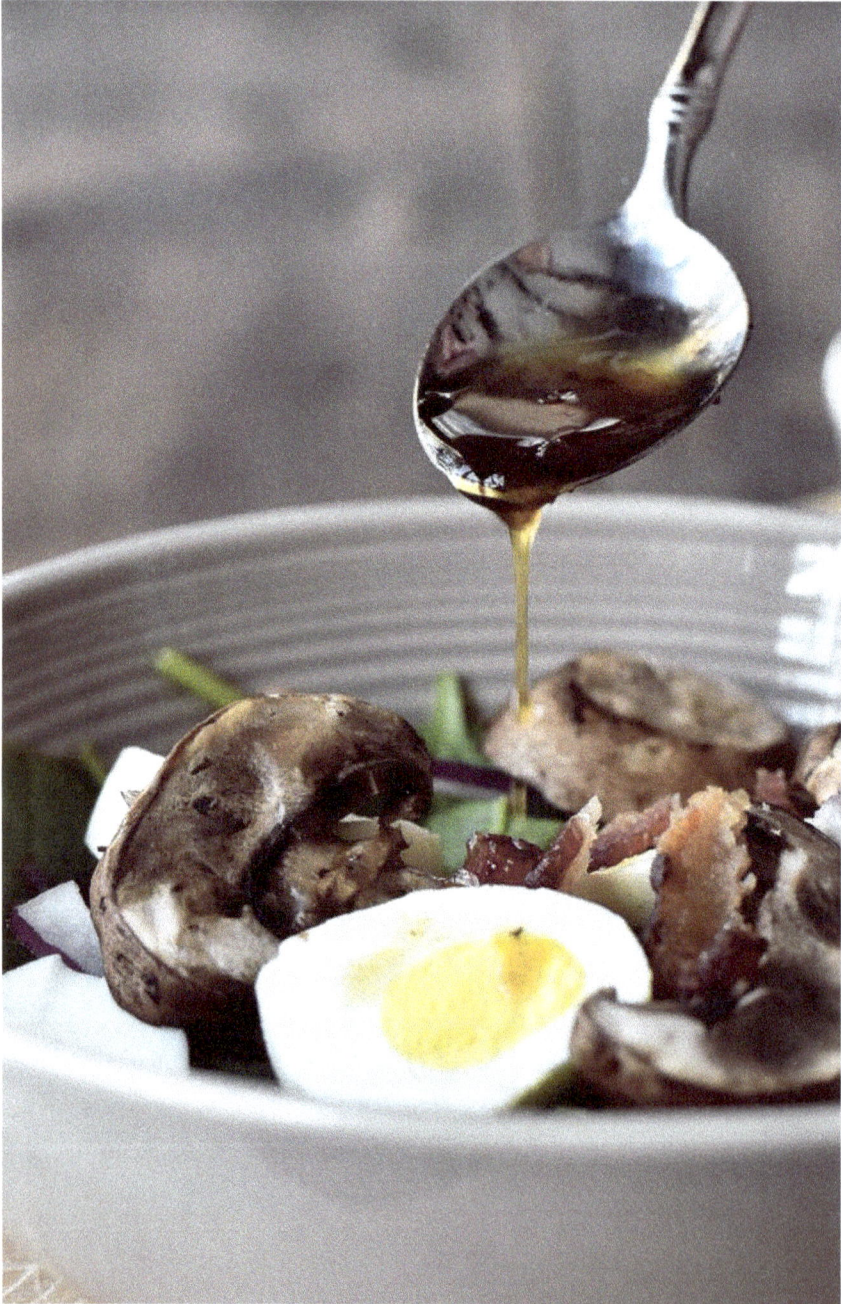

Preparation Time: 15 Minutes

Cooking Time: 0 Minutes

Servings: 4

Ingredients

- 8 slices center-cut bacon
- 3 tbsp. extra virgin olive oil
- 1 (5-oz) pkg baby spinach
- 1 tbsp. apple cider vinegar
- 1 tsp. Dijon mustard
- 1/2 tsp. honey
- 1/4 tsp. salt
- 1/2 tsp. pepper

Directions:

1. Mix vinegar, mustard, honey, salt and pepper in a bowl.

2. Whisk in oil. Place spinach in a serving bowl; drizzle with dressing, and toss to coat.

3. Sprinkle with cooked and crumbled bacon.

Nutrition:

Calories 110

Protein 6 g

Fat 2 g

Carbs 1 g

Pea and Collards Soup

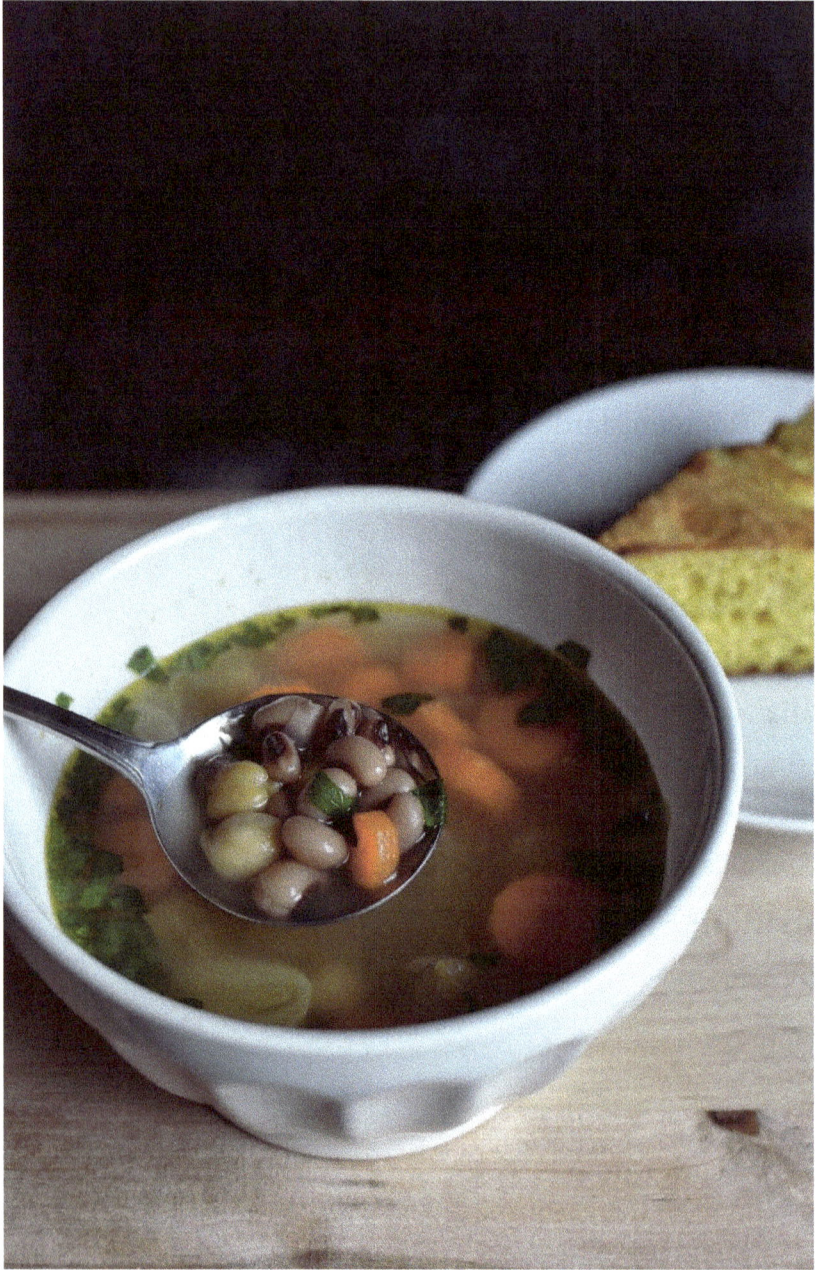

Preparation Time: 10 Minutes

Cooking Time: 30 Minutes

Servings: 4

Ingredients

- 1/2 (16-oz) pkg black-eyed peas

- 1 onion

- 2 carrots

- 1,5 cups ham (low-sodium)

- 1 (1-lb) bunch collard greens (trimmed)

- 1 tbsp. extra virgin olive oil

- 2 cloves garlic

- 1/2 tsp. black pepper

- Hot sauce

Directions:

1. Cook chopped onion and carrots 10 Minutes.

2. Add peas, diced ham, collards, and Minced garlic. Cook 5 Minutes.

3. Add broth, 3 cups water, and pepper. Bring to a boil; simmer 35 Minutes, adding water if needed.

Serve with favorite sauce.

Nutrition:

Calories 86

Protein 15 g

Fat 2 g

Carbs 9 g

Spanish Stew

Preparation Time: 10 Minutes

Cooking Time: 25 Minutes

Servings: 4

Ingredients

- **1.** 1/2 (12-oz) pkg smoked chicken sausage links

- 1 (5-oz) pkg baby spinach

- 1 (15-oz) can chickpeas

- 1 (14. 5-oz) can tomatoes with basil, garlic, and oregano

- 1/2 tsp. smoked paprika

- 1/2 tsp. cumin

- 3/4 cup onions

- 1 tbsp. extra virgin olive oil

Directions:

1. Cook sliced the sausage in hot oil until browned. Remove from pot.

2. Add chopped onions; cook until tender.

3. Add sausage, drained and rinsed chickpeas, diced tomatoes, paprika, and ground cumin. Cook 15 Minutes.

4. Add in spinach; cook 1 to 2 Minutes.

This dish is ideal for every day and for a festive table.

Nutrition:

Calories 200

Protein 10 g

Fat 20 g

Carbs 1 g

Creamy Taco Soup

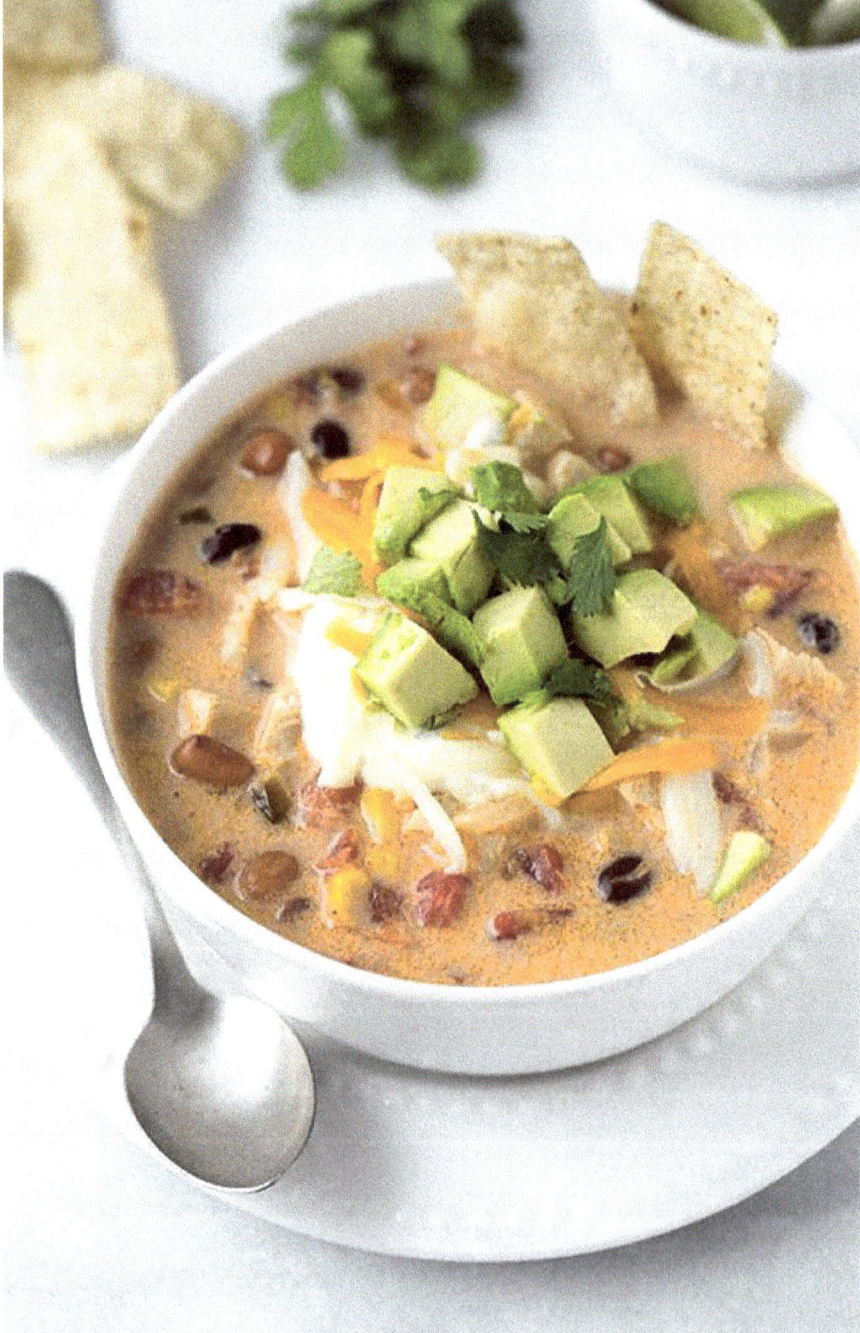

Preparation Time: 10 Minutes

Cooking Time: 20 Minutes

Servings: 4

Ingredients

- 3/4 lb. ground sirloin
- 1/2 (8-oz) cream cheese
- 1/2 onion
- 1 clove garlic
- 1 (10-oz) can tomatoes and green chiles
- 1 (14. 5-oz) can beef broth
- 1/4 cup heavy cream
- 1,5 tsp. cumin
- 1/2 tsp. chili powder

Directions:

1. Cook beef, chopped onion, and Minced garlic until meat is browned and crumbly; drain and return to pot.

2. Add ground cumin, chili powder, and cream cheese cut into small pieces and softened, stirring until cheese is melted.

3. Add diced tomatoes, broth, and cream; bring to a boil, and simmer 10 Minutes. Season with pepper and salt to taste.

You've got to give someone the recipe for this soup dish!

Nutrition:

Calories 60

Protein 3 g

Fat 1 g

Carbs 8 g

Chicken with Caprese Salsa

Preparation Time: 15 Minutes

Cooking Time: 5 Minutes

Servings: 4

Ingredients

- 3/4 lb. boneless, skinless chicken breasts

- 2 big tomatoes

- 1/2 (8-oz) ball fresh mozzarella cheese

- 1/4 cup red onion

- 2 tbsp. fresh basil

- 1 tbsp. balsamic vinegar

- 2 tbsp. extra virgin olive oil (divided)

- 1/2 tsp. salt (divided)

- 1/4 tsp. pepper (divided)

Directions:

1. Sprinkle cut in half lengthwise chicken with 1/4 tsp. salt and 1/8 tsp. pepper.

2. Heat 1 tbsp. olive oil, cook chicken 5 Minutes.

3. Meanwhile, mix chopped tomatoes, diced cheese, finely chopped onion, chopped basil, vinegar, 1 tbsp. oil, and 1/4 tsp. salt and 1/8 tsp. pepper.

4. Spoon salsa over chicken.

Chicken with Caprese Salsa is a nutritious, simple and very tasty dish that can be prepared in a few Minutes.

Nutrition:

Calories 210

Protein 28 g

Fat 17 g

Carbs 0, 1 g

Balsamic-Roasted Broccoli

Preparation Time: 10 Minutes

Cooking Time: 15 Minutes

Servings: 4

Ingredients

- 1 lb. broccoli
- 1 tbsp. extra virgin olive oil
- 1 tbsp. balsamic vinegar
- 1 clove garlic
- 1/8 tsp. salt
- Pepper to taste

Directions

1. Preheat oven to 450F.

2. Combine broccoli, olive oil, vinegar, Minced garlic, salt, and pepper; toss.

3. Spread broccoli on a baking sheet.

4. Bake 12 to 15 Minutes.

5. Really good!

Nutrition:

Calories 27

Protein 3 g

Fat 0, 3 g

Carbs 4 g

Hearty Beef And Vegetable Soup

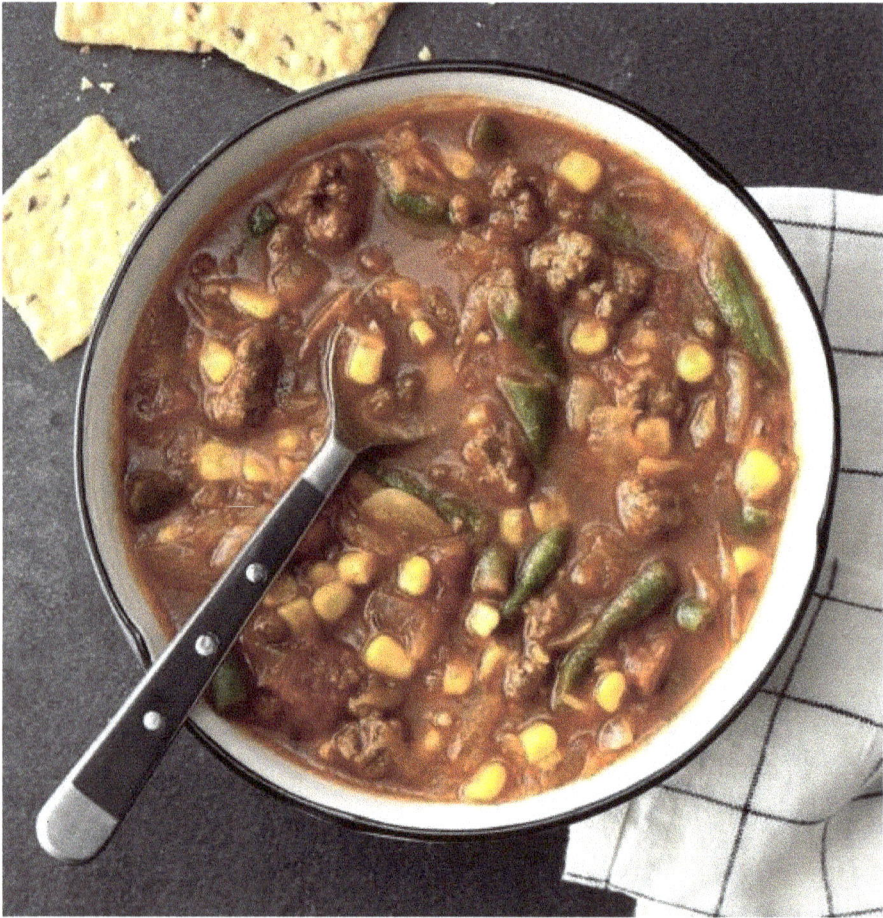

Preparation Time: 10 Minutes

Cooking Time: 30 Minutes

Servings: 4

Ingredients

- 1/2 lb. lean ground beef
- 2 cups beef broth
- 1,5 tbsp. vegetable oil (divided)
- 1 cup green bell pepper
- 1/2 cup red onion
- 1 cup green cabbage
- 1 cup frozen mixed vegetables
- 1/2 can tomatoes
- 1,5 tsp. Worcestershire sauce
- 1 small bay leaf
- 1,8 tsp. pepper
- 2 tbsp. ketchup

Directions:

1. Cook beef in 1/2 tbsp. hot oil 2 Minutes.

2. Stir in chopped bell pepper and chopped onion; cook 4 Minutes.

3. Add chopped cabbage, mixed vegetables, stewed tomatoes, broth, Worcestershire sauce, bay leaf, and pepper; bring to a boil.

4. Reduce heat to medium; cover, and cook 15 Minutes.

5. Stir in ketchup and 1 tbsp. oil, and remove from heat. Let stand 10 Minutes.

The right diet is excellent diabetes remedy.

Nutrition:

Calories 170

Protein 17 g

Fat 8 g

Carbs 3 g

Cauliflower Muffin

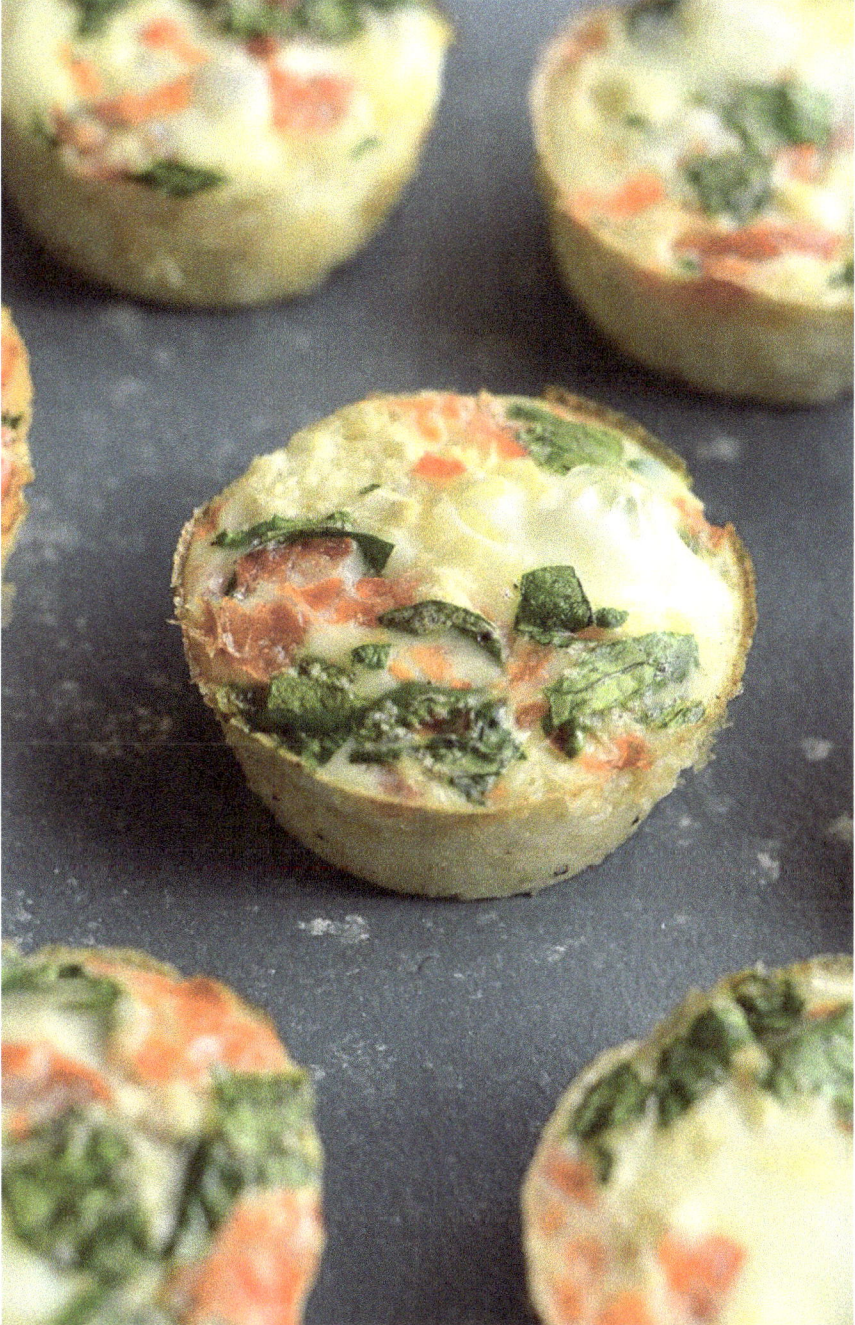

Preparation Time: 15 Minutes

Cooking Time: 30 Minutes

Servings: 4

Ingredients

- 2,5 cup cauliflower
- **Servings:** cup ham
- 2,5 cups of cheese
- **Servings:** cup champignon
- 1,5 tbsp. flaxseed
- 3 eggs
- 1/4 tsp. salt
- 1/8 tsp. pepper

Directions:

1. Preheat oven to 375 F.

2. Put muffin liners in a 12-muffin tin.

3. Combine diced cauliflower, ground flaxseed, beaten eggs, cup diced ham, grated cheese, and diced mushrooms, salt, pepper.

4. Divide mixture rightly between muffin liners.

5. Bake 30 Minutes.

This is a great lunch for the whole family.

Nutrition:

Calories 116

Protein 10 g

Fat 7 g

Carbs 3 g

Ham And Egg Cups

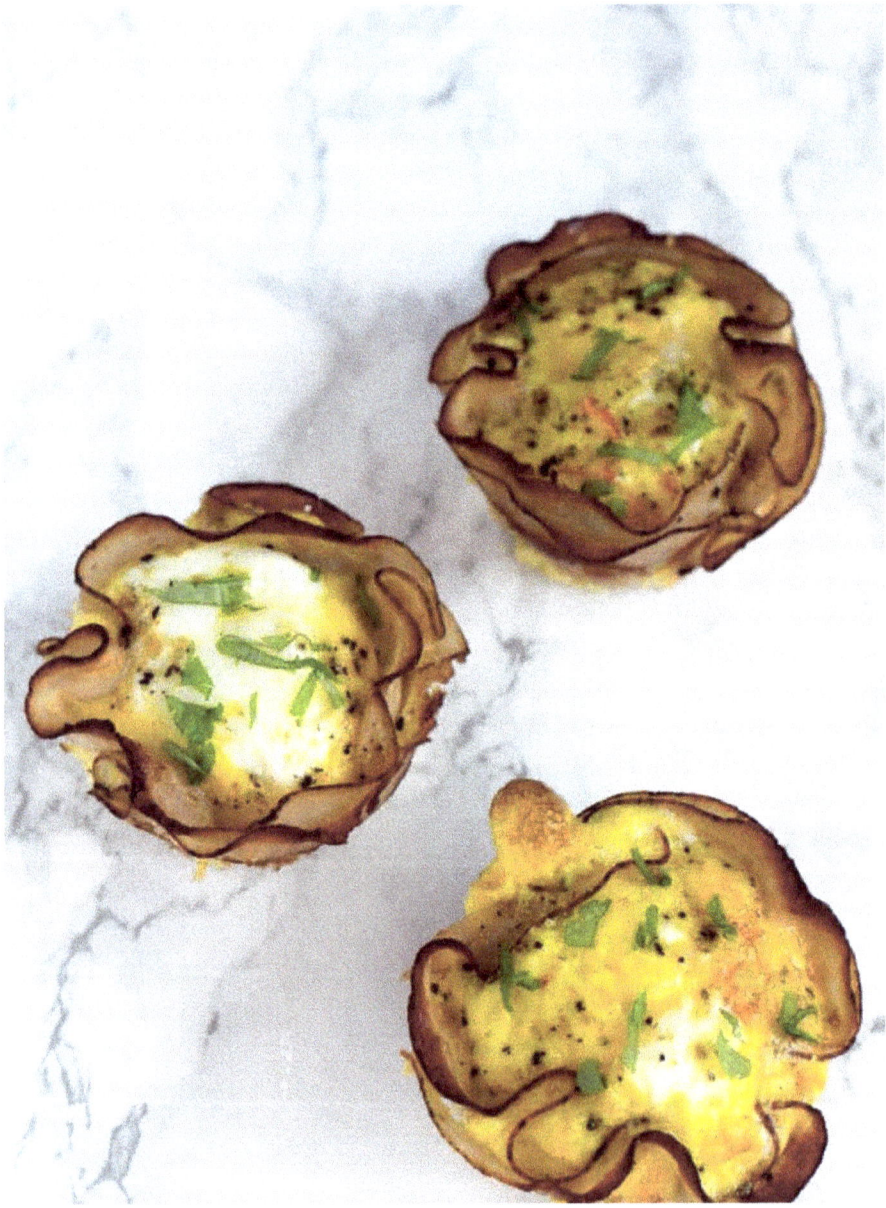

Preparation Time: 10 Minutes

Cooking Time: 15 Minutes

Servings: 4

Ingredients

- 5 slices ham
- 4 tbsp. cheese
- 1,5 tbsp. cream
- 3 egg whites
- 1,5 tbsp. pepper (green)
- 1 tsp. salt
- pepper to taste

Directions:

1. Preheat oven to 350 F.

2. Arrange each slice of thinly sliced ham into 4 muffin tin.

3. Put 1/4 of grated cheese into ham cup.

4. Mix eggs, cream, salt and pepper and divide it into 2 tins.

5. Bake in oven 15 Minutes; after baking, sprinkle with green onions.

If you want to keep your current shape, also pay attention to this dish.

Nutrition:

Calories 180

Protein 13 g

Fat 13 g

Carbs 2 g

Cauliflower Rice With Chicken

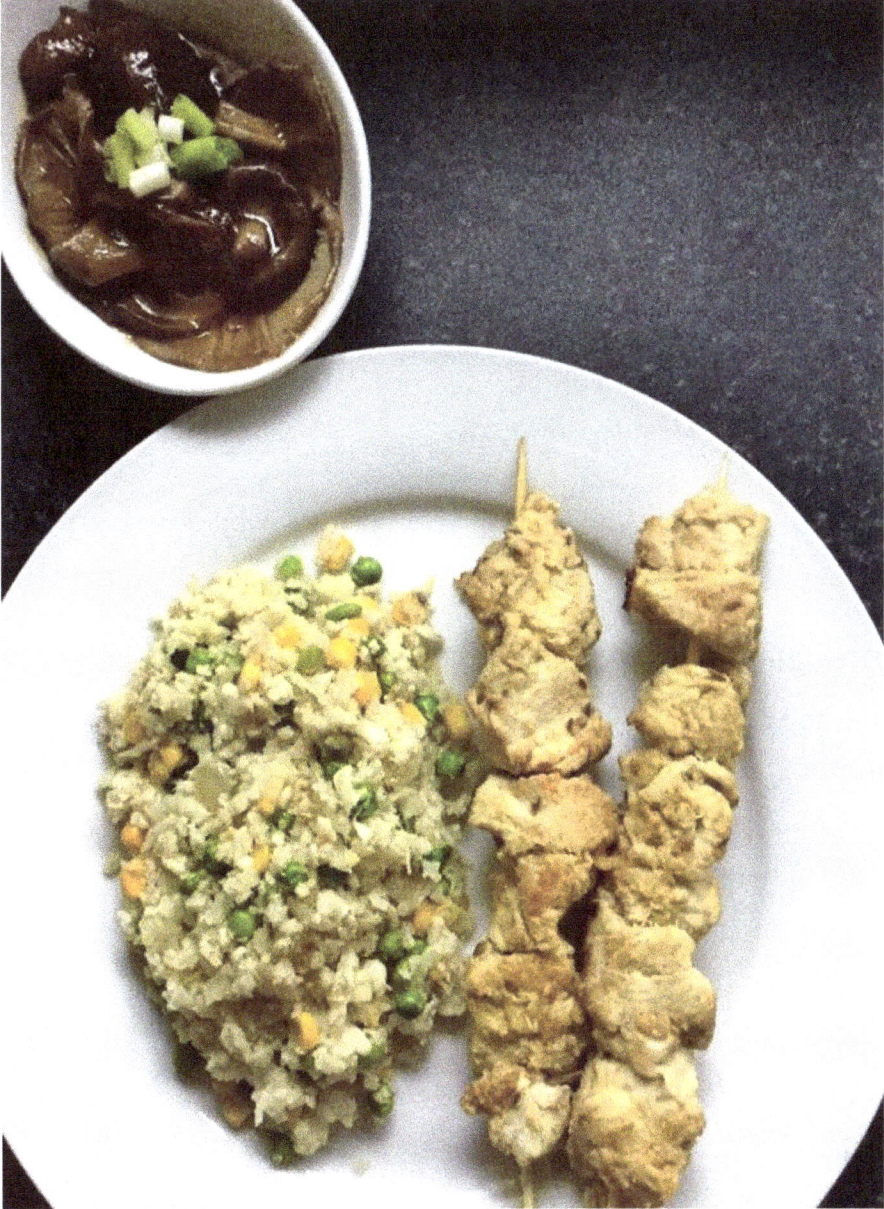

Preparation Time: 15 Minutes

Cooking Time: 15 Minutes

Servings: 4

Ingredients

- 1/2 large cauliflower
- 3/4 cup cooked meat
- 1/2 bell pepper
- 1 carrot
- 2 ribs celery
- 1 tbsp. stir fry sauce (low carb)
- 1 tbsp. extra virgin olive oil
- Salt and pepper to taste

Directions:

1. Chop cauliflower in a processor to "rice." Place in a bowl.

2. Properly chop all vegetables in a food processor into thin slices.

3. Add cauliflower and other plants to WOK with heated oil. Fry until all veggies are tender.

4. Add chopped meat and sauce to the wok and fry 10 Minutes.

Serve.

This dish is very mouth-watering!

Nutrition:

Calories 200

Protein 10 g

Fat 12 g

Carbs 10 g

Turkey With Fried Eggs

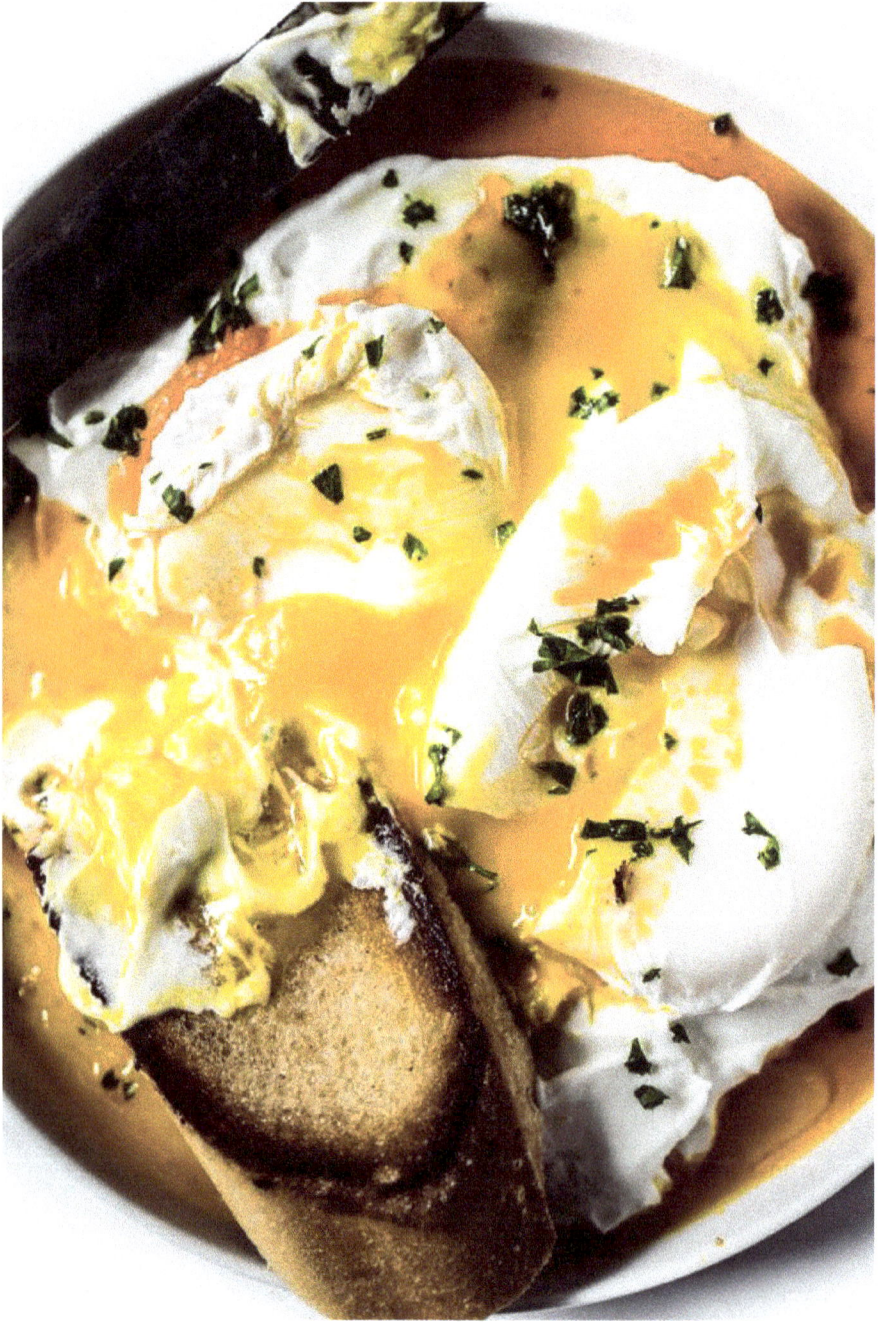

Preparation Time: 10 Minutes

Cooking Time: 20 Minutes

Servings: 4

Ingredients

- 4 large potatoes

- 1 cooked turkey thigh

- 1 large onion (about 2 cups diced)

- butter

- Chile flakes

- 4 eggs

- salt to taste

- pepper to taste

Directions:

1. Rub the cold boiled potatoes on the coarsest holes of a box grater. Dice the turkey.

2. Cook the onion in as much unsalted butter as you feel comfortable with until it's just fragrant and translucent.

3. Add the rubbed potatoes and a cup of diced cooked turkey, salt and pepper to taste, and cook 20 Minutes.

Top each with a fried egg. Yummy!

Nutrition:

Calories 170

Protein 19 g

Fat 7 g

Carbs 6 g

Sweet Potato, Kale, And White Bean Stew

Preparation Time: 15 minutes

Cooking Time: 25 minutes

Servings: 4

Ingredients :

• 1 (15-ounce) can low-sodium cannellini beans, rinsed and drained, divided

• 1 tablespoon olive oil

• 1 medium onion, chopped

• 2 garlic cloves, minced

• 2 celery stalks, chopped

• 3 medium carrots, chopped

• 2 cups low-sodium vegetable broth

• 1 teaspoon apple cider vinegar

• 2 medium sweet potatoes (about 1¼ pounds)

• 2 cups chopped kale

• 1 cup shelled edamame

• ¼ cup quinoa

• 1 teaspoon dried thyme

• 1/2 teaspoon cayenne pepper

• 1/2 teaspoon salt

• ¼ teaspoon freshly ground black pepper

Directions:

1. Put half the beans into a blender and blend until smooth. Set aside.

2. In a large soup pot over medium heat, heat the oil. When the oil is shining, include the onion and garlic, and cook until the onion softens and the garlic is sweet, about 3 minutes. Add the celery and carrots, and continue cooking until the vegetables soften, about 5 minutes.

3. Add the broth, vinegar, sweet potatoes, unblended beans, kale, edamame, and quinoa, and bring the mixture to a boil. Reduce the heat and simmer until the vegetables soften, about 10 minutes.

4. Add the blended beans, thyme, cayenne, salt, and black pepper, increase the heat to medium-high, and bring the mixture to a boil. Reduce the heat and simmer, uncovered, until the flavors combine, about 5 minutes.

5. Into each of 4 containers, scoop 1¾ cups of stew.

Nutrition:

calories: 373;

total fat: 7g;

saturated fat: 1g;

protein: 15g;

total carbs: 65g;

fiber: 15g;

sugar: 13g;

sodium: 540mg

Lighter Eggplant Parmesan

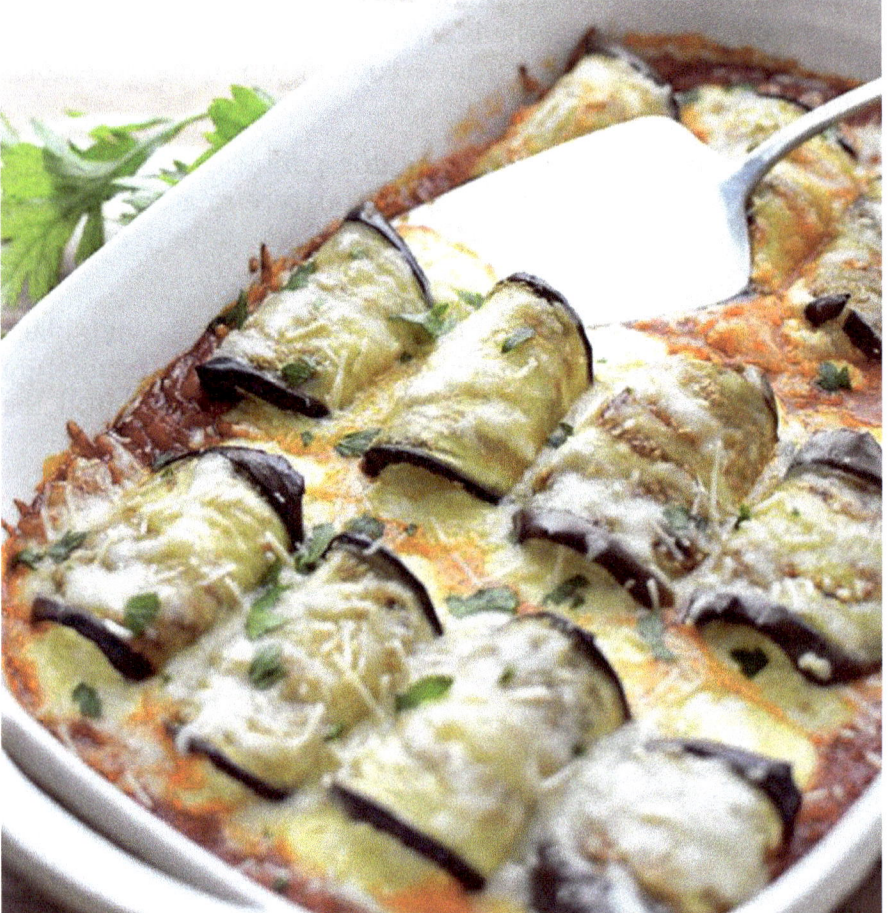

Preparation Time: 15 minutes

Cooking Time: 35 minutes

Servings: 4

Ingredients :

• Nonstick cooking spray

• 3 eggs, beaten

• 1 tablespoon dried parsley

- 2 teaspoons ground oregano

- 1/8 teaspoon freshly ground black pepper

- 1 cup panko bread crumbs, preferably whole-wheat

- 1 large eggplant (about 2 pounds)

- 5 servings (21/2 cups) chunky tomato sauce or jarred low-sodium tomato sauce

- 1 cup part-skim mozzarella cheese

- ¼ cup grated parmesan cheese

Directions:

1. Preheat the oven to 450f. Coat a baking sheet with cooking spray.

2. In a medium bowl, whisk together the eggs, parsley, oregano, and pepper.

3. Pour the panko into a separate medium bowl.

4. Slice the eggplant into ¼-inch-thick slices. Dip each slice of eggplant into the egg mixture, shaking off the excess. Then dredge both sides of the eggplant in the panko bread crumbs. Place the coated eggplant on the prepared baking sheet, leaving a 1/2-inch space between each slice.

5. Bake for about 15 minutes until soft and golden brown. Remove from the oven and set aside to slightly cool.

6. Pour 1/2 cup of chunky tomato sauce on the bottom of an 8-by-15-inch baking dish. Using a spatula or the back of a spoon spread the tomato sauce evenly. Place half the slices of cooked eggplant, slightly overlapping, in the dish, and top with 1 cup of chunky tomato sauce, 1/2 cup of mozzarella and 2 tablespoons of grated parmesan. Repeat the layer, ending with the cheese.

7. Bake uncovered for 20 minutes until the cheese is bubbling and slightly browned.

8. Remove from the oven and allow cooling for 15 minutes before dividing the eggplant equally into 4 separate containers.

Nutrition:

calories: 333;

total fat: 14g;

saturated fat: 6g;

protein: 20g;

total carbs: 35g;

fiber: 11g;

sugar: 15g;

sodium: 994mg

Coconut-Lentil Curry

Preparation Time: 15 minutes

Cooking Time: 35 minutes

Servings: 4

Ingredients :

• 1 tablespoon olive oil

• 1 medium yellow onion, chopped

• 1 garlic clove, minced

• 1 medium red bell pepper, diced

• 1 (15-ounce) can green or brown lentils, rinsed and drained

• 2 medium sweet potatoes, washed, peeled, and cut into bite-size chunks (about 1¼ pounds)

• 1 (15-ounce) can no-salt-added diced tomatoes

• 2 tablespoons tomato paste

• 4 teaspoons curry powder

• 1/8 teaspoon ground cloves

• 1 (15-ounce) can light coconut milk

• ¼ teaspoon salt

• 2 pieces whole-wheat naan bread, halved, or 4 slices crusty bread

Directions:

1. In a large saucepan over medium heat, heat the olive oil. When the oil is shimmering, add both the onion and garlic and cook until the onion softens and the garlic is sweet, for about 3 minutes.

2. Add the bell pepper and continue cooking until it softens, about 5 minutes more. Add the lentils, sweet potatoes, tomatoes, tomato paste, curry powder, and cloves, and bring the mixture to a boil. Reduce the heat to medium-low, cover, and simmer until the potatoes are softened, about 20 minutes.

3. Add the coconut milk and salt, and return to a boil. Reduce the heat and simmer until the flavors combine, about 5 minutes.

4. Into each of 4 containers, spoon 2 cups of curry.

5. Enjoy each serving with half of a piece of naan bread or 1 slice of crusty bread.

Nutrition:

calories: 559;

total fat: 16g;

saturated fat: 7g;

protein: 16g;

total carbs: 86g;

fiber: 16g;

sugar: 18g;

sodium: 819mg

Stuffed Portobello With Cheese

Preparation Time: 15 minutes

Cooking Time: 25 minutes

Servings: 4

Ingredients :

• 4 Portobello mushroom caps

• 1 tablespoon olive oil

• 1/2 teaspoon salt, divided

• ¼ teaspoon freshly ground black pepper, divided

• 1 cup baby spinach, chopped

• 11/2 cups part-skim ricotta cheese

• 1/2 cup part-skim shredded mozzarella cheese

• ¼ cup grated parmesan cheese

• 1 garlic clove, minced

• 1 tablespoon dried parsley

• 2 teaspoons dried oregano

• 4 teaspoons unseasoned bread crumbs, divided

• 4 servings (4 cups) roasted broccoli with shallots

Directions:

1. Preheat the oven to 375f. Line a baking sheet with aluminum foil.

2. Brush the mushroom caps with the olive oil, and sprinkle with ¼ teaspoon salt and 1/8 teaspoon pepper. Put the mushroom caps on the prepared baking sheet and bake until soft, about 12 minutes.

3. In a medium bowl, mix together the spinach, ricotta, mozzarella, parmesan, garlic, parsley, oregano, and the remaining ¼ teaspoon of salt and 1/8 teaspoon of pepper.

4. Spoon 1/2 cup of cheese mixture into each mushroom cap, and sprinkle each with 1 teaspoon of bread crumbs. Return the mushrooms to the oven for an additional 8 to 10 minutes until warmed through.

5. Remove from the oven and allow the mushrooms to cool for about 10 minutes before placing each in an individual container. Add 1 cup of roasted broccoli with shallots to each container.

Nutrition:

calories: 419;

total fat: 30g;

saturated fat: 10g;

protein: 23g;

total carbs: 19g;

fiber: 2g;

sugar: 3g;

sodium: 790mg

Lighter Shrimp Scampi

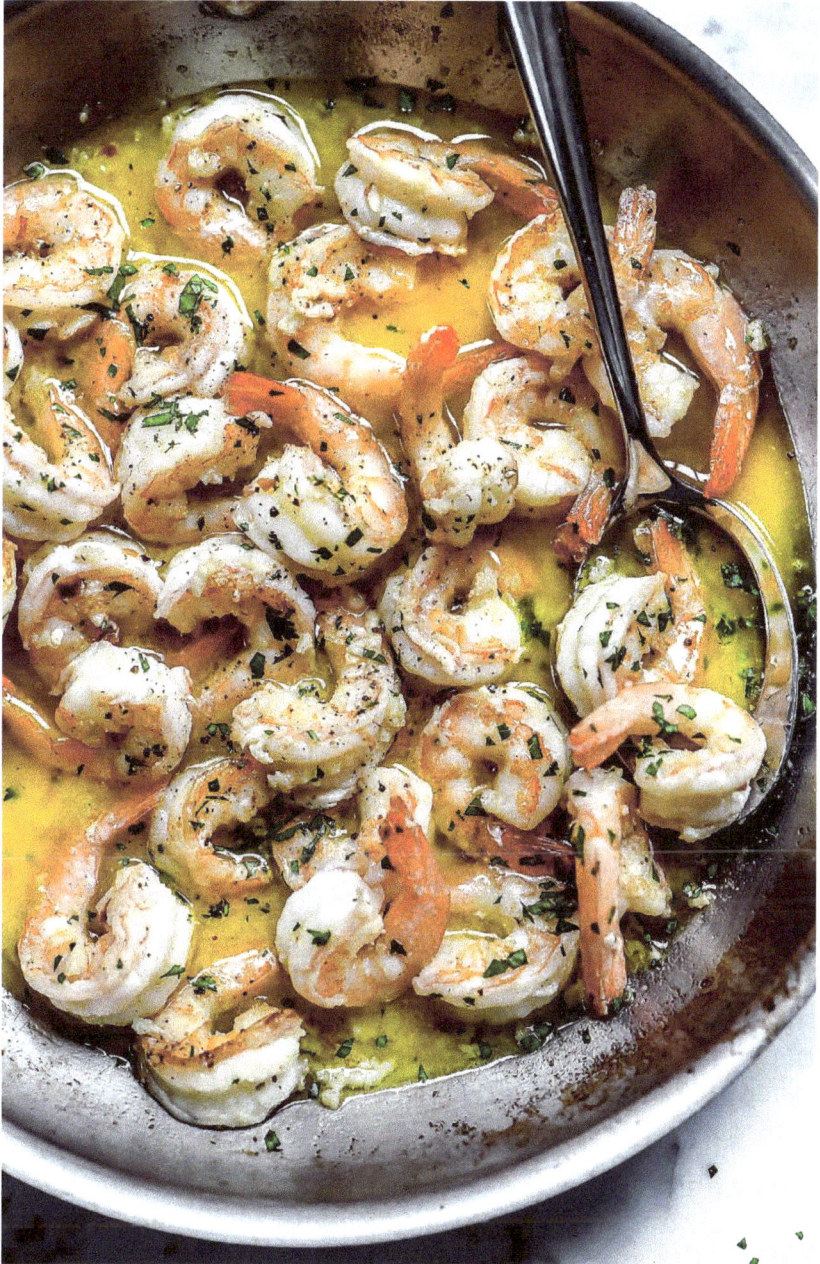

Preparation Time: 15 minutes

Cooking Time: 15 minutes

Servings: 4

Ingredients :

• 11/2 pounds large peeled and deveined shrimp

• ¼ teaspoon salt

• 1/8 teaspoon freshly ground black pepper

• 2 tablespoons olive oil

• 1 shallot, chopped

• 2 garlic cloves, minced

• ¼ cup cooking white wine

• Juice of 1/2 lemon (1 tablespoon)

• 1/2 teaspoon sriracha

• 2 tablespoons unsalted butter, at room temperature

• ¼ cup chopped fresh parsley

• 4 servings (6 cups) zucchini noodles with lemon vinaigrette

Directions:

1. Season the shrimp with the salt and pepper.

2. In a medium saucepan over medium heat, heat the oil. Add the shallot and garlic, and cook until the shallot softens and the garlic is fragrant, about 3 minutes. Add the shrimp, cover, and cook until opaque, 2 to 3 minutes on each side. Using a slotted spoon, transfer the shrimp to a large plate.

3. Add the wine, lemon juice, and sriracha to the saucepan, and stir to combine. Bring the mixture to a boil, then reduce the heat and simmer until the liquid is reduced by about half, 3 minutes. Add the butter and stir until melted, about 3 minutes. Return the shrimp to the saucepan and toss to coat. Add the parsley and stir to combine.

4. Into each of 4 containers, place 11/2 cups of zucchini noodles with lemon vinaigrette, and top with ¾ cup of scampi.

Nutrition:

calories: 364;

total fat: 21g;

saturated fat: 6g;

protein: 37g;

total carbs: 10g;

fiber: 2g;

sugar: 6g;

sodium: 557mg

Maple-Mustard Salmon

Preparation Time: 10 minutes, plus 30 minutes marinating time

Cooking Time: 20 minutes

Servings: 4

Ingredients :

• Nonstick cooking spray

• 1/2 cup 100% maple syrup

• 2 tablespoons Dijon mustard

• ¼ teaspoon salt

• 4 (5-ounce) salmon fillets

• 4 servings (4 cups) roasted broccoli with shallots

• 4 servings (2 cups) parsleyed whole-wheat couscous

Directions:

1. Preheat the oven to 400f. Line a baking sheet with aluminum foil and coat with cooking spray.

2. In a medium bowl, whisk together the maple syrup, mustard, and salt until smooth.

3. Put the salmon fillets into the bowl and toss to coat. Cover and place in the refrigerator to marinate for at least 30 minutes and up to overnight.

4. Shake off excess marinade from the salmon fillets and place them on the prepared baking sheet, leaving a 1-inch space between each fillet. Discard the extra marinade.

5. Bake for about 20 minutes until the salmon is opaque and a thermometer inserted in the thickest part of a fillet reads 145f.

6. Into each of 4 resealable containers, place 1 salmon fillet, 1 cup of roasted broccoli with shallots, and 1/2 cup of parsleyed whole-wheat couscous.

Nutrition:

calories: 601;

total fat: 29g;

saturated fat: 4g;

protein: 36g;

total carbs: 51g;

fiber: 3g;

sugar: 23g;

sodium: 610mg

Chicken Salad With Grapes And Pecans

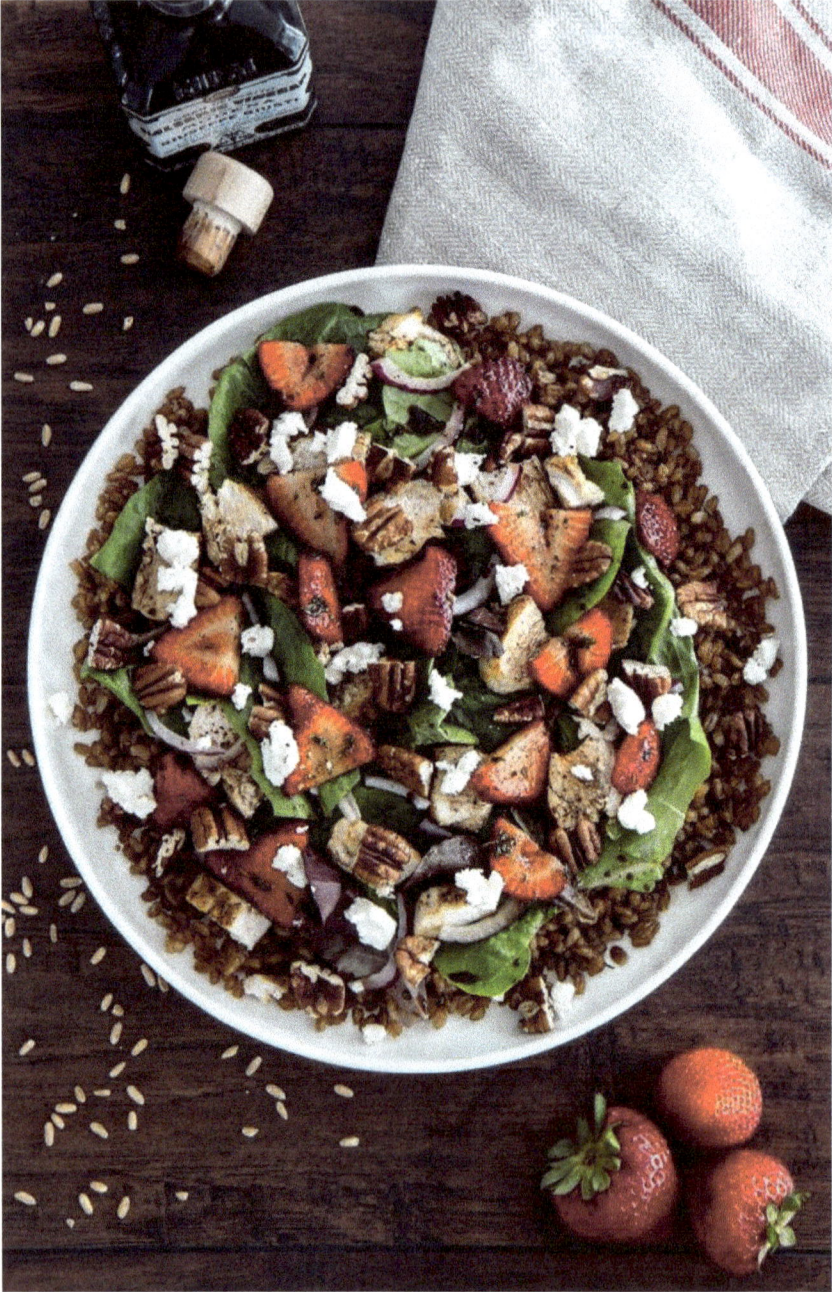

Preparation Time: 15 Minutes

Cooking Time: 5 Minutes

Servings: 4

Ingredients :

• 1/3 cup unsalted pecans, chopped

• 10 ounces cooked skinless, boneless chicken breast or rotisserie chicken, finely chopped

• 1/2 medium yellow onion, finely chopped

• 1 celery stalk, finely chopped

• ¾ cup red or green seedless grapes, halved

• ¼ cup light mayonnaise

• ¼ cup nonfat plain Greek yogurt

• 1 tablespoon Dijon mustard

• 1 tablespoon dried parsley

• ¼ teaspoon salt

• 1/8 teaspoon freshly ground black pepper

• 1 cup shredded romaine lettuce

• 4 (8-inch) whole-wheat pitas

Directions:

1. Heat a small skillet over medium-low heat to toast the pecans. Cook the pecans until fragrant, about 3 minutes. Remove from the heat and set aside to cool.

2. In a medium bowl, mix the chicken, onion, celery, pecans, and grapes.

3. In a small bowl, whisk together the mayonnaise, yogurt, mustard, parsley, salt, and pepper. Spoon the sauce over the chicken mixture and stir until well combined.

4. Into each of 4 containers, place ¼ cup of lettuce and top with 1 cup of chicken salad. Store the pitas separately until ready to serve.

5. When ready to eat, stuff the serving of salad and lettuce into 1 pita.

Nutrition:

Calories: 418;

Total Fat: 14g;

Saturated Fat: 2g;

Protein: 31g;

Total Carbs: 43g;

Fiber: 6g;

Courgettes In Cider Sauce

Preparation Time: 13 minutes

Cooking Time: 17 minutes

Servings: 3

Ingredients :

• 2 cups baby courgettes

• 3 tablespoons vegetable stock

• 2 tablespoons apple cider vinegar

• 1 tablespoon light brown sugar

• 4 spring onions, finely sliced

• 1 piece fresh gingerroot, grated

• 1 teaspoon corn flour

• 2 teaspoons water

Directions:

1. Bring a pan with salted water to a boil. Add courgettes. Bring to a boil for 5 minutes.

2. Meanwhile, in a pan, combine vegetable stock, apple cider vinegar, brown sugar, onions, gingerroot, lemon juice and rind, and orange juice and rind. Take to a boil. Lower the heat and allow simmering for 3 minutes.

3. Mix the corn flour with water. Stir well. Pour into the sauce. Continue stirring until the sauce thickens.

4. Drain courgettes. Transfer to the serving dish. Spoon over the sauce. Toss to coat courgettes. Serve.

Nutrition:

Calories 173

Total Fat 9. 2 g

Saturated Fat 0.8 g

Cholesterol 0 mg

Sodium 861 mg

Total Carbs 22. 5 g

Fiber 6. 3 g

Sugar 2. 3 g

Protein 9. 2 g

Baked Mixed Mushrooms

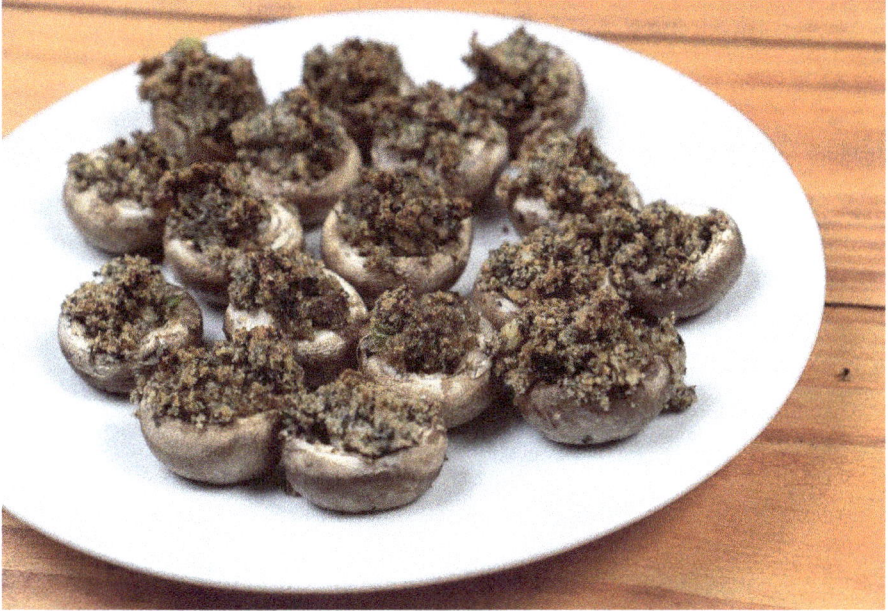

Preparation Time: 8 minutes

Cooking Time: 20 minutes

Servings: 3

Ingredients :

- 2 cups mixed wild mushrooms
- 1 cup chestnut mushrooms
- 2 cups dried porcini
- 2 shallots
- 4 garlic cloves
- 3 cups raw pecans
- ½ bunch fresh thyme
- 1 bunch flat-leaf parsley

- 2 tablespoons olive oil

- 2 fresh bay leaves

- 1 ½ cups stale bread

Directions:

1. Remove skin and finely chop garlic and shallots. Roughly chop the wild mushrooms and chestnut mushrooms. Pick the leaves of the thyme and tear the bread into small pieces. Put inside the pressure cooker.

2. Place the pecans and roughly chop the nuts. Pick the parsley leaves and roughly chop.

3. Place the porcini in a bowl then add 300ml of boiling water. Set aside until needed.

4. Heat oil in the pressure cooker. Add the garlic and shallots. Cook for 3 minutes while stirring occasionally.

5. Drain porcini and reserve the liquid. Add the porcini into the pressure cooker together with the wild mushrooms and chestnut mushrooms. Add the bay leaves and thyme.

6. Position the lid and lock in place. Put to high heat and bring to high pressure. Adjust heat to stabilize. Cook for 10 minutes. Adjust taste if necessary.

7. Transfer the mushroom mixture into a bowl and set aside to cool completely.

8. Once the mushrooms are completely cool, add the bread, pecans, a pinch of black pepper and sea salt, and half of the reserved liquid into the bowl. Mix well. Add more reserved liquid if the mixture seems dry.

9. Add more than half of the parsley into the bowl and stir. Transfer the mixture into a 20cm x 25cm lightly greased baking dish and cover with tin foil.

10. Bake in the oven for 35 minutes. Then, get rid of the foil and cook for another 10 minutes. Once done, sprinkle the remaining parsley on top and serve with bread or crackers. Serve.

Nutrition:

Calories 343

Total Fat 4. 2 g

Saturated Fat 0.8 g

Cholesterol 0 mg

Sodium 861 mg

Total Carbs 22. 5 g

Fiber 6. 3 g

Sugar 2. 3 g

Protein 9. 2 g

Alkaline Buns Recipe

Preparation Time: 20 minutes

Cooking Time: 40 minutes

Servings: 6

Ingredients :

- 2 1/4 cups - 2 1/2 cups spelt flour

- 1/2 cup hemp milk or walnut milk

- 1/4 cup aquafaba

- 1/4 cup sparkling spring water

- 1 tbsp. Agave

- 1 tbsp. Onion powder

- 1 1/2 tsp. Sea salt

- 1 tsp. Basil or oregano

- 2 tsp. Grapeseed oil

- 1 tsp. Sea moss gel (optional)

- Sesame seeds (optional)

- Mixer with dough hook*

- Baking sheet

- Plastic wrap

- Parchment paper

- Note: if you do not have a mixer, you can knead by hand.

Directions:

1. Add all the dry Ingredients into a mixing bowl and blend perfectly.

2. Add the remaining Ingredients and blend on low speed for a minute. Then, knead dough at medium speed for 5 minutes.

3. Sprinkle grapeseed oil on a baking sheet already laced with parchment paper.

4. Separate dough into parts, roll with hand to make shapes then place on baking sheet.

5. Brush the top with oil then add sesame seeds.

6. Use a plastic wrap to cover the buns and allow it to sit for 30 minutes.

7. Set your oven to 350°f and bake for 30 minutes.

8. Allow the buns to cook and carefully cut them in half to enjoy your alkaline electric buns!

Nutrition:

Carbohydrates: 47 grams

Fat: 7 grams

Protein: 9 grams

Alkaline Strawberry Jam Recipe

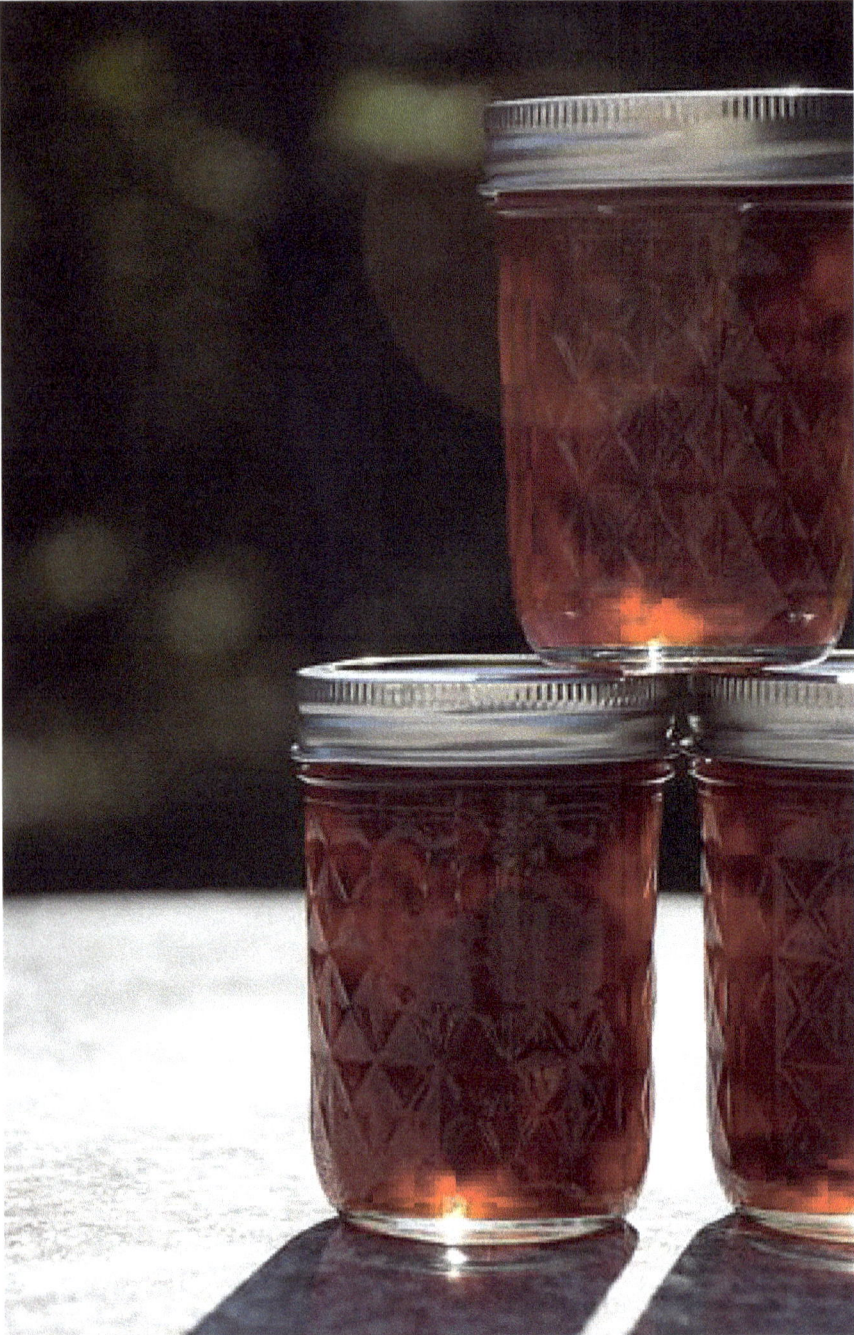

Preparation Time: 10 minutes

Cooking Time: 20 minutes

Servings: 16 oz

Ingredients :

- 4 cups sliced strawberries
- **Servings:** cups of raw agave
- 3 tablespoons of key lime juice
- 1/2 cup irish moss gel

Directions:

1. Slice enough strawberries to fill up 4 cups.

2. Mash or blend to your desired texture.

3. Agave, lime juice and strawberries should be added to the sauce pan on high heat.

4. Cook for 10 minutes then add irish moss gel.

5. Cook for 5 more minutes to make certain that the gel has been thoroughly dissolved.

6. Remove from heat and allow the saucc to cool down before refrigerating.

7. Dish your alkaline electric strawberry jam!

Nutrition:

Calories: 56

Carbohydrate: 13 grams

Alkaline Date Syrup Recipe

Preparation Time: 10 minutes

Cooking Time: 15 minutes

Servings: 16-24 oz

Ingredients :

• 1 cup dates, preferably pitted

• 1 cup of spring water

• This sweetener can be easily dissolved in water unlike date sugar.

Directions:

1. Boil spring water then remove from heat when boiled.

2. Place dates in the boiled water for at least 5 minutes.

3. Pour the dates and some water into a blender then blend for until it's smooth.

4. If the texture is too thick, add more water and blend again.

5. Keep it a refrigerator and dish with alkaline date syrup!

Nutrition:

Calories: 270

Potassium: 848 milligrams

Sodium: 5 milligrams

Carbohydrates: 67 grams

Fiber: 3 grams

Sugar: 61 grams

Protein: 1 grams

Chickpea Mashed Potatoes

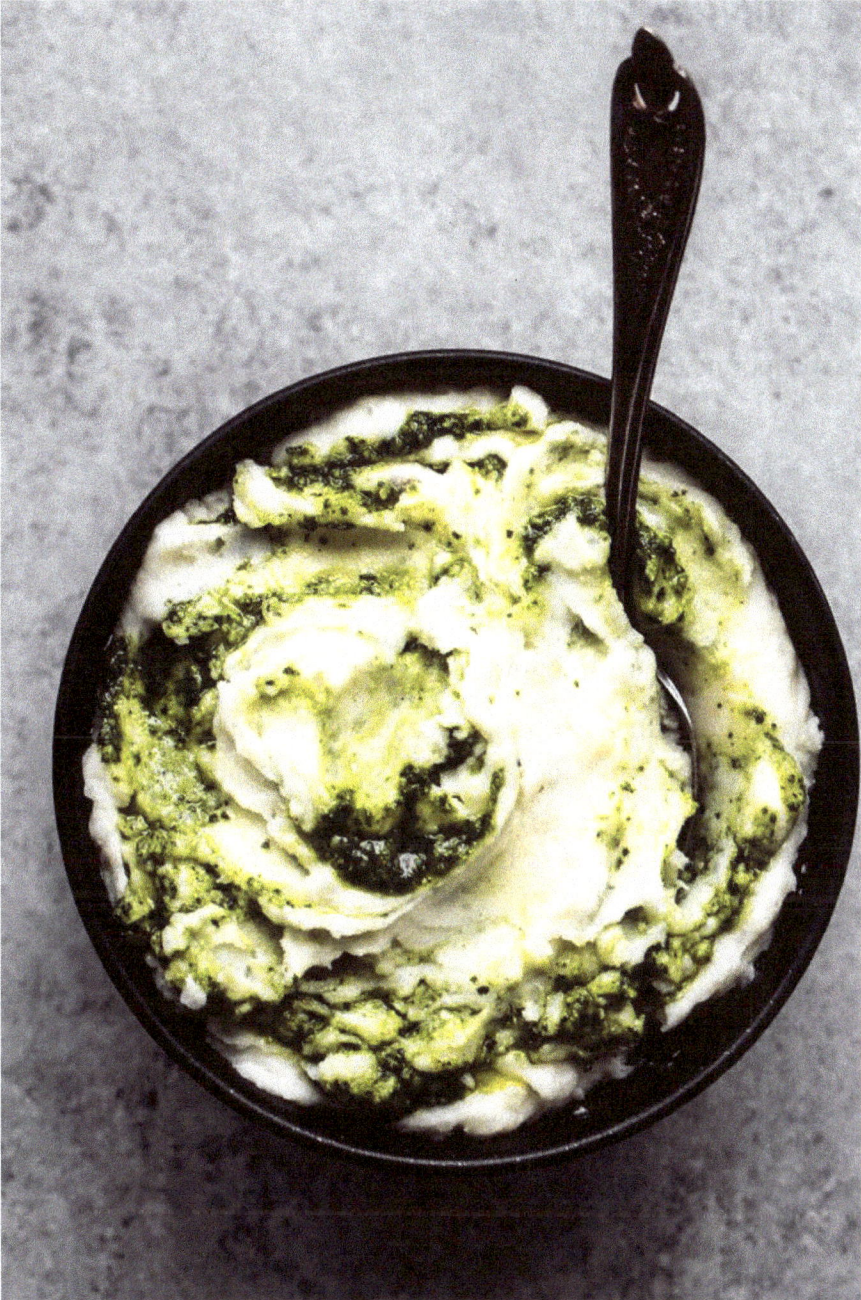

Preparation Time: 5 minutes

Cooking Time: 30 minutes

Servings: 4

Ingredients :

• 2 cups chickpeas, cooked

• ¼ cup green onions, diced

• 2 teaspoons sea salt

• 2 teaspoons onion powder

• 1 cup walnut milk; homemade, unsweetened

Directions:

1. Plug in a food processor, add chickpeas to it, pour in the milk, and then add salt and onion powder.

2. Cover the blending jar with its lid and then pulse for 1 to 2 minutes until smooth; blend in water if the mixture is too thick.

3. Take a medium saucepan, place it over medium heat, and then add blended chickpea mixture in it.

4. Stir green onions into the chickpeas mixture and then cook the mixture for 30 minutes, stirring constantly.

5. Serve straight away.

Nutrition:

Calories: 145.8

Carbohydrates: 19.1 grams

Fat: 7.3 grams

Protein: 3.3 grams

Mushroom And Onion Gravy

Preparation Time: 5 minutes

Cooking Time: 18 minutes

Servings: 4

Ingredients :

- 1 cup sliced onions, chopped
- 1 cup mushrooms, sliced
- 2 teaspoons onion powder
- 2 teaspoons sea salt
- 1 teaspoon dried thyme
- 6 tablespoons chickpea flour
- ½ teaspoon cayenne pepper
- 1 teaspoon dried oregano
- 4 tablespoons grapeseed oil
- 4 cups spring water

Directions:

1. Take a medium pot, place it over medium-high heat, add oil and when hot, add onions and mushrooms, and then cook for 1 minute.

2. Season the vegetables with onion powder, salt, thyme, and oregano. Stir until mixed, and cook for 5 minutes.

3. Pour in water, stir in cayenne pepper, stir well, and then bring the mixture to a boil.

4. Slowly stir in chickpea flour, and bring the mixture to a boil again.

5. Remove pan from heat and then serve gravy with a favorite dish.

Nutrition:

Calories: 120

Carbohydrates: 8.4 grams

Fat: 7.6 grams

Protein: 2.2 grams

Vegetable Chili

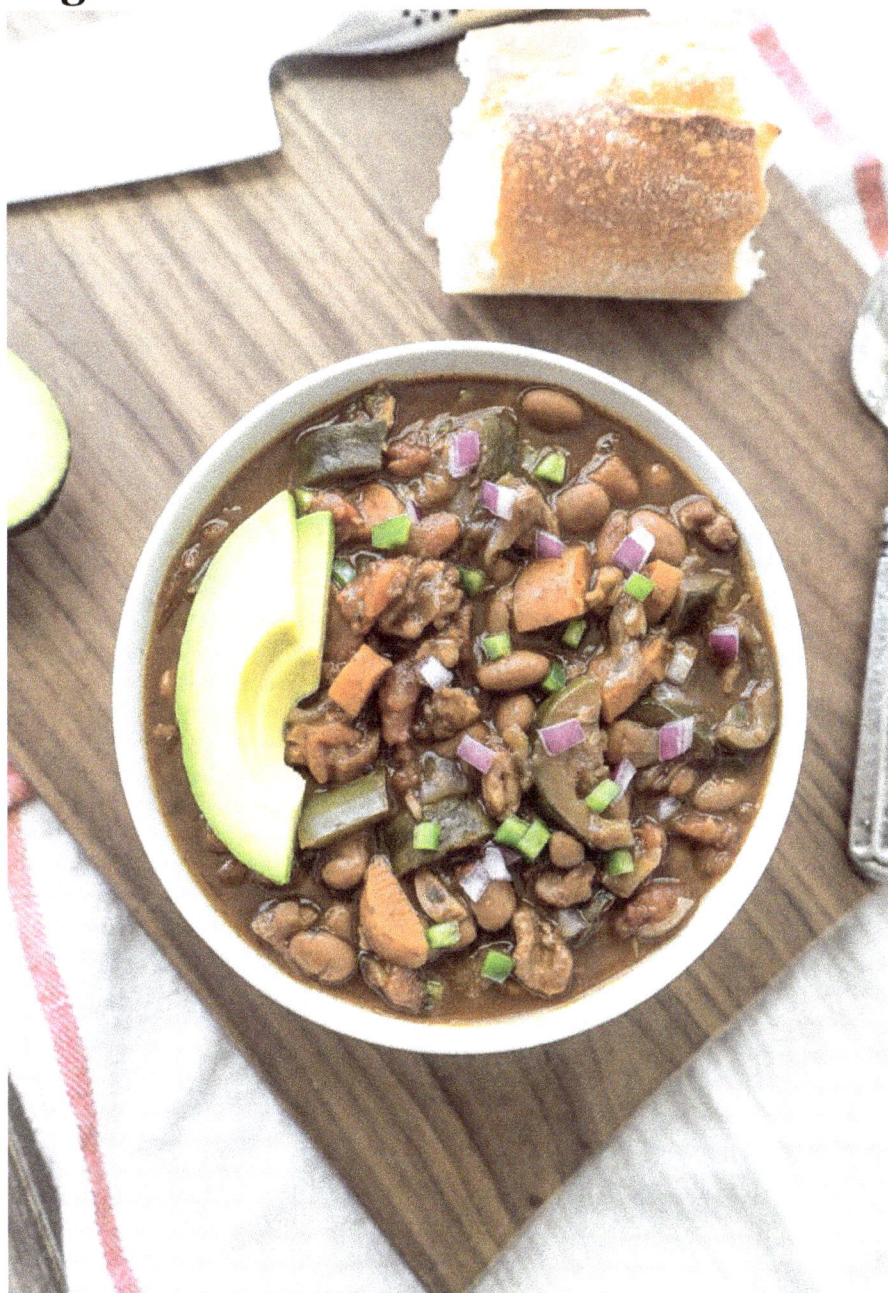

Preparation Time: 5 minutes

Cooking Time: 30 minutes

Servings: 6

Ingredients :

• 2 cups black beans, cooked

• 1 medium red bell pepper; deseeded, chopped

• 1 poblano chili; deseeded, chopped

• 2 jalapeño chilies; deseeded, chopped

• 4 tablespoons cilantro, chopped

• 1 large white onion; peeled, chopped

• 1 ½ tablespoon minced garlic

• 1 ½ teaspoon sea salt

• 1 ½ teaspoon cumin powder

• 1 ½ teaspoon red chili powder

• 3 teaspoons lime juice

• 2 tablespoons grapeseed oil

• 2 ½ cups vegetable stock

Directions:

1. Take a large pot, place it over medium-high heat, add oil and when hot, add onion and cook for 4–5 minutes until translucent.

2. Add bell pepper, jalapeno pepper, poblano chili, and garlic and then cook for 3–4 minutes until veggies turn tender.

3. Season the vegetables with salt, stir in cumin powder and red chili powder, then add chickpeas and pour in vegetable stock.

4. Bring the mixture to a boil, then switch heat to

medium-low and simmer the chili for 15–20 minutes

until thickened slightly.

5. Then remove the pot from heat, ladle chili stew among six bowls, drizzle with lime juice, garnish with cilantro, and serve.

Nutrition:

Calories: 224.2

Carbs: 42.6 grams

Fat: 1.2 grams

Protein: 12.5 grams.

www.ingramcontent.com/pod-product-compliance
Lightning Source LLC
Chambersburg PA
CBHW050756030426
42336CB00012B/1845